Demos Surgical Pathology Guides

Inflammatory Skin Disorders

SERIES EDITOR

Saul Suster, MD
Professor and Chairman
Department of Pathology
Medical College of Wisconsin
Milwaukee, Wisconsin

TITLES

- *Head and Neck Pathology*
  Paul E. Wakley

- *Breast Pathology*
  Giovanni Falconieri, Janez Lamovec, and Abiy B. Ambaye

FORTHCOMING TITLES

- *Skin Tumors*
  Jose A. Plaza and Victor G. Prieto

- *Pulmonary Pathology*
  R. Nagarjun Rao and Cesar A. Moran

- *Soft Tissues*
  Eduardo V. Zambrano

- *Lymph Nodes*
  Steven H. Kroft, Alexandra Harrington, and Horatiu Olteanu

- *Gastrointestinal Pathology*
  Richard A. Komorowski

Demos Surgical Pathology Guides

Inflammatory Skin Disorders

JOSE A. PLAZA, MD
Director of Dermatopathology
Medical College of Wisconsin and Froedtert Hospital
Milwaukee, Wisconsin

VICTOR G. PRIETO, MD, PHD
Director of Dermatopathology
MD Anderson Cancer Center
Houston, Texas

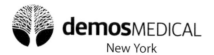
New York

ISBN: 978-1-933864-87-7
ebook ISBN: 978-1-935281-96-2

Acquisitions Editor: Rich Winters
Compositor: S4Carlisle Publishing Services

Visit our website at www.demosmedpub.com

Medicine is an ever-changing science. Research and clinical experience are continually expanding our knowledge, in particular our understanding of proper treatment and drug therapy. The authors, editors, and publisher have made every effort to ensure that all information in this book is in accordance with the state of knowledge at the time of production of the book. Nevertheless, the authors, editors, and publisher are not responsible for errors or omissions or for any consequences from application of the information in this book and make no warranty, express or implied, with respect to the contents of the publication. Every reader should examine carefully the package inserts accompanying each drug and should carefully check whether the dosage schedules mentioned therein or the contraindications stated by the manufacturer differ from the statements made in this book. Such examination is particularly important with drugs that are either rarely used or have been newly released on the market.

Library of Congress Cataloging-in-Publication Data
Plaza, Jose A.
  Inflammatory skin disorders / Jose A. Plaza, Victor G. Prieto.
    p. ; cm. — (Demos surgical pathology guides)
  Includes bibliographical references and index.
  ISBN-13: 978-1-933864-87-7
  ISBN-10: 1-933864-87-7
  ISBN-13: 978-1-935281-96-2 (ebook)
  ISBN-10: 1-935281-96-8 (ebook)
  I. Prieto, Victor G. II. Title. III. Series: Demos surgical pathology guides.
    [DNLM: 1. Skin Diseases—pathology. 2. Diagnosis, Differential. 3. Inflammation.
    4. Skin Diseases—diagnosis. WR 140]
  616.5—dc23
                                                                    2011038898

Special discounts on bulk quantities of Demos Medical Publishing books are available to corporations, professional associations, pharmaceutical companies, health care organizations, and other qualifying groups. For details, please contact:

Special Sales Department
Demos Medical Publishing
11 W. 42nd Street, 15th Floor
New York, NY 10036
Phone: 800–532–8663 or 212–683–0072
Fax: 212–941–7842
E-mail: rsantana@demosmedpub.com

Printed in the United States of America at Bradford & Bigelow.
12 13 14 15 5 4 3 2 1

Contents

Series Foreword

The field of surgical pathology has gained increasing relevance and importance over the years as pathologists have become more and more integrated into the health care team. To the need for precise histopathologic diagnoses has now been added the burden of providing our clinical colleagues with information that will allow them to assess the prognosis of the disease and predict the response to therapy. Pathologists now serve as key consultants in the patient management team and are responsible for providing critical information that will guide their therapy. With the progress gained due to the insights obtained from the application of newer diagnostic techniques, surgical pathology has become progressively more complex. As a result, diagnoses need to be more detailed and specific and the number of data elements required in the generation of a surgical pathology report have increased exponentially, making management of the information required for diagnosis cumbersome and sometimes difficult.

The past 15 years have witnessed an explosion of information in the field of pathology with a massive proliferation of specialized textbooks appearing in print. For the most part, such texts provide in-depth and detailed coverage of the various areas in surgical pathology. The purpose of this series is to bridge the gap between the major subspecialty texts and the large, double-volume general surgical pathology textbooks, by providing compact, single-volume monographs that will succinctly address the most salient and important points required for the diagnosis of the most common conditions. The series is organized following an organ-system format, with single volumes dedicated to individual organs. The volumes are divided on the basis of disease groups, including benign reactive, inflammatory, infectious or systemic conditions, benign neoplastic conditions, and malignant neoplasms. Each chapter consists of a bulleted list of the most pertinent clinical data related to the condition, followed by the most important histopathologic criteria for diagnosis, pertinent use of immunohistochemical stains and other ancillary techniques, and relevant molecular tests when available. This is followed by a section on differential diagnosis. References appear at the back of the volume. Each entity is illustrated with key, high-quality histological images that highlight the most salient and distinctive features that need to be recognized for the correct diagnosis.

These books are intended for the busy practicing pathologist, and for pathology residents and fellows in training who require an easy and simple overview of major diagnostic criteria and key points during the course of routine daily practice. The authors have been carefully chosen for their experience in the field and clarity of exposition in the various topics. It is hoped that this series will fulfill its purpose of providing quick and easy access to critical information for the busy practitioner or trainee, and that it will assist pathologists in their routine practice of the specialty.

Saul Suster, MD
Professor and Chairman
Department of Pathology
Medical College of Wisconsin
Milwaukee, Wisconsin

Preface

At first glance, pathologists and dermatologists may interpret the histologic analysis of inflammatory conditions in the skin as extremely complicated. A good number of diseases may show similar histopathologic features. Many of those diseases evolve, thus showing different histologic features depending at what moment on the evolution of the disease the biopsy is taken. And, as in other fields, the histopathologist has to rely on the amount and quality of the clinical information provided by the clinician taking the biopsy.

Despite all the above-described problems, in most cases the histopathologist can establish either the definite diagnosis (e.g., psoriasis, herpetic dermatitis) or else provide a histologic pattern that will aid the clinician to diagnose the disease (e.g., interface dermatitis with superficial and deep perivascular infiltrate of lymphocytes and plasma cells, in a patient with positive anti-nuclear antibodies is most likely cutaneous lupus erythematosus). This volume will describe the major patterns of skin inflammatory conditions along with the most common entities included in each differential diagnosis. The two main features for proper classification are the distribution of the inflammatory infiltrate (superficial, deep, interstitial, band-like in the epidermis and dermis; lobular or septal in the subcutaneous tissue) and its cellular composition (neutrophils, eosinophils, lymphocytes, macrophages, and melanophages). Since it is relatively common that features of more than one pattern are present in a single biopsy, the histopathologist should determine which pattern is the most prominent and then proceed to establish the appropriate differential diagnosis.

HISTOLOGIC PATTERNS:

Inflammatory reactions mostly involving the epidermis:
- **Spongiotic** (intercellular edema in the epidermis = spongiosis)
- **Psoriasiform** (elongation of the rete ridges with cellular infiltrates in the papillary dermis. It may be accompanied by spongiosis)

- **Lichenoid/interface** (linear arrangement of lymphocytes in the papillary dermis, also along the dermal–epidermal junction). As others, we consider lichenoid dermatitis as part of *interface dermatitis* (i.e., a process that involves the dermal–epidermal region regardless of the amount of inflammatory cells)
- **Blistering** (Presence of a cleft. It is subclassified according to the level of the split: subcorneal, intraepidermal, suprabasal, subepidermal, dermal)

Inflammatory reactions primarily involving the dermis:
- **Interstitial** (dermal infiltrate among collagen bundles)
- **Vasculopathic** (dermal infiltrate involving the dermal blood vessels with damage to the vessel wall. When it reaches frank destruction it is labeled vasculitis)
- **Fibrosing** (increased amounts of collagen in the dermis)

Inflammatory reactions primarily involving the subcutaneous tissue:
- **Panniculitis** (inflammatory infiltrate in the subcutaneous tissue)

Cutaneous deposition disorders:
- **Dermal mucinoses** (increased amount of mucin)
- **Other cutaneous deposition disorders** (crystals, calcium, amyloid, etc.)

Inflammatory Reactions Primarily Limited to the Epidermis

1

SPONGIOTIC DERMATITIS (ECZEMA)
CONTACT DERMATITIS
ATOPIC DERMATITIS
NUMMULAR ECZEMA
DYSHIDROTIC ECZEMA
ID REACTION (AUTOSENSITIZATION)
SEBORRHEIC DERMATITIS

OTHER FORMS OF SPONGIOTIC DERMATITIS
PITYRIASIS ROSEA
STASIS DERMATITIS

PSORIASIFORM DERMATITIS
PSORIASIS
LICHEN SIMPLEX CHRONICUS
PITYRIASIS RUBRA PILARIS
REITER SYNDROME
PELLAGRA
ACRODERMATITIS ENTEROPATHICA
NECROLYTIC MIGRATORY ERYTHEMA (GLUCAGONOMA)
NECROLYTIC ACRAL ERYTHEMA

SPONGIOTIC DERMATITIS (ECZEMA)

Spongiotic dermatitis is a descriptive name for a group of skin conditions that clinically manifest as an erythematous and papulovesicular eruption. As the condition progress into the chronic phase, they appear as thickened (lichenoid) plaques. The spongiotic reaction is characterized by intraepidermal and intercellular edema (spongiosis) and is histologically recognized by the widened intercellular spaces between keratinocytes, with elongation of the intercellular bridges. Since spongiotic dermatitides are insufficiently distinct on histologic grounds to separate them into more specific categories, our recommendation is to sign-out these cases with a descriptive terminology, i.e., "spongiotic dermatitis," along with a microscopic description. Spongiotic dermatitis can be subdivided into three different phases: acute, subacute, and chronic.

HISTOLOGY:

- **Acute Phase:** The stratum corneum has an intact pattern (basket-weave). The epidermis shows accumulation of fluid (spongiosis). Also, formation of microvesicles due to rupture of desmosomal attachments is characteristic at this stage. Mild papillary dermal edema and lymphocytic exocytosis can be seen. In the superficial dermis there is mild perivascular lymphocytic infiltrates sometimes admixed with eosinophils (especially in contact dermatitis).
- **Subacute Phase:** The epidermis tends to be more acanthotic and hyperplastic along with areas of parakeratosis. The granular layer may be diminished. At this stage, the epidermis shows less spongiosis and less edema in the dermis.
- **Chronic Phase:** The stratum corneum shows hyperkeratosis with or without parakeratosis. The epidermis shows acanthosis and hyperplasia with only minimal spongiosis (psoriasiform hyperplasia may be evident). The granular layer tends to be thickened. The papillary dermis is fibrous with a patchy lymphocytic infiltrate. Spongiotic dermatitis, especially in the chronic phase, may be difficult to separate from psoriasis given the psoriasiform epidermal hyperplasia.

VARIATIONS:

Contact Dermatitis

Contact dermatitis can be subdivided into allergic and irritant types. Allergic contact dermatitis is a type-IV (cellular) hypersensitivity that is initiated by contact with an allergen to which the person has previously been sensitized, such as latex or poison ivy (1). Irritant contact dermatitis results from direct damage to the epidermis from the causative agent, e.g., detergents, solvents, acids, etc. (2). Histologically, both show spongiotic changes. A histologic characteristic for the diagnosis of allergic contact dermatitis is the predominance of eosinophils and the presence of Langerhans cell microabscesses within the epidermis (sometimes called eosinophilic spongiosis). However, these changes are not entirely specific since they can be seen, among others, in bullous pemphigoid and incontinentia pigmenti (3, 4) (**Figure 1-1A, B**) (**Table 1-1**).

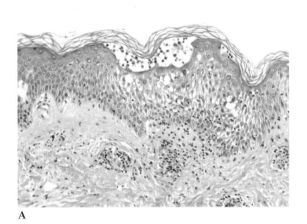 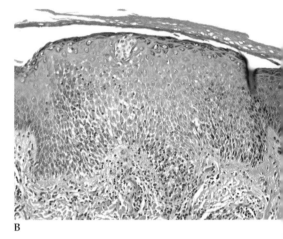

A   B

FIGURE 1-1
A. *Subacute spongiotic dermatitis* (allergic contact dermatitis). Epidermal acanthosis with spongiosis and Langerhans cell microvesicles. **B.** *Spongiotic dermatitis.* Hyperkeratosis, acanthosis, spongiosis with lymphocytic exocytosis. A small Langerhans cell microvesicle is present in the epidermis. This case also represents an example of allergic contact dermatitis.

Atopic Dermatitis

Atopic dermatitis is a common eczematous condition that is commonly related to a family history of atopy (hay fever, allergic rhinitis, asthma, dry skin and increased levels of IgE) (5). In infants the lesions are more commonly seen around the face, in children the lesions commonly involve the flexural areas (anticubital and popliteal) and in adults the presentation is variable. It tends to fade during childhood, but it can present lifelong exacerbations during adolescence or adulthood. The histologic features will depend on the stage of the lesion; however, there is often follicular accentuation of the lymphocytic infiltrate, prominence of small blood vessels in the papillary dermis, atrophy of sebaceous glands (especially in patients with ichthyosis vulgaris) and epidermal acanthosis with partial psoriasiform folding (6, 7).

Nummular Dermatitis

Nummular dermatitis is characterized by coin-shaped, round, vesicular, crusted, and usually pruritic lesions more commonly seen on the dorsum of the hands, forearms and legs. The pathophysiology is unknown but several factors have been suggested (8). Clinically, it can be confused with dermatophytosis and granuloma annulare. Histologically, the lesions will mirror the evolution of other spongiotic processes.

Dyshidrotic Eczema

Dyshidrotic eczema (pompholyx) is a recurrent or chronic relapsing form of vesicular and itchy palmoplantar dermatitis (9). The etiology of dyshidrotic eczema is unknown but it appears to be related to other skin diseases including atopic dermatitis, contact dermatitis, allergy to ingested metals, dermatophyte infection, bacterial infection, environmental or emotional stress, etc. (10). Histologically, there are intraepidermal spongiotic vesicles or bullae. In dermis, there is a lymphocytic infiltrate with neutrophils focally involving the epidermis (**Figure 1-2**). It is always recommended to perform a PAS to rule out fungal organisms.

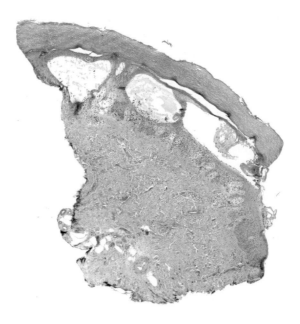

FIGURE 1-2 *Dyshidrotic Eczema (Pompholyx)*
Large intraepidermal spongiotic vesicles filled with rare neutrophils.

Id Reaction (Autosensitization)

Id reaction is a pruritic, eczematous dermatitis that is associated with, but usually distant to, another skin lesion that could be either an inflammatory or an infectious condition. The most common inciting conditions associated with reactions include dermatophytosis (usually tinea pedis) and stasis dermatitis. Histologically, the biopsies will show spongiotic changes.

Seborrheic Dermatitis

Usually it affects areas of the skin that are rich in sebaceous glands and sebum, such as scalp, eyebrows, eyelids, paranasal folds, axilla, etc. The condition is characterized clinically by "greasy," scaly and red to brown patches (11). Seborrheic dermatitis is one of the most common cutaneous manifestations seen in the acquired immunodeficiency syndrome (AIDS) (12). It is also seen with increased frequency in association in other diseases such as Parkinson disease, obesity, etc. (13). The histologic features are similar to the other causes of eczematous dermatitis, but in addition the early phase will show more exocytosis of neutrophils and mononuclear cells; Pityrosporum yeasts may be noted in the stratum corneum. In chronic phase, follicles will show ostia with follicular plugging, lateral parakeratosis and a scale crust with neutrophils (**Figure 1-3**). When related to AIDS it may show scattered apoptotic keratinocytes and plasma cells in dermis (14).

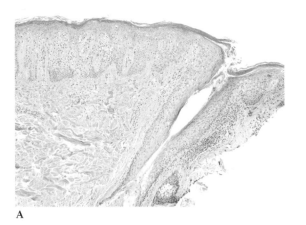
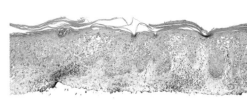

A   B

FIGURE 1-3 *Seborrheic Dermatitis*
A. Spongiotic and acanthotic epidermis with mild parakeratosis at the follicular ostia.
B. Spongiotic epidermis with acanthosis and parakeratosis with some neutrophilic exocytosis.

TABLE 1-1 Differential Diagnosis of Eosinophilic Spongiosis (**Figure 1-4**)

Allergic contact dermatitis
Drug eruptions
Urticarial phase of bullous pemphigoid
Arthropod bite reactions
Early phase of pemphigus
Incontinentia pigmenti (early stage)

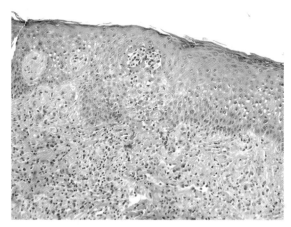

FIGURE 1-4 *Eosinophilic Spongiosis*
Epidermis with spongiosis and an increased number of eosinophils in both epidermis and dermis. This case is an example of a drug reaction.

There are many other dermatoses that show spongiotic changes on histology and may have additional, characteristic features to allow a specific diagnosis.

Pityriasis Rosea

Pityriasis rosea (PR) is a common, self-limited dermatitis that affects mainly children and young adults. PR is similar to infectious exanthems in that it occurs in clusters among contacts, has a seasonal predilection and may have an infectious (viral) etiology (i.e., herpes virus 6 and 7 [HHV-6 & HHV-7]) (15). Clinically, the skin rash usually appears as a single oval scaly patch, the "herald patch," particularly on the trunk followed by pink widespread patches (on the trunk and proximal extremities) often in a linear arrangement resembling a "Christmas tree" (16).

HISTOLOGY (FIGURE 1-5):
- Mounds of skipping parakeratosis in the stratum corneum
- Diminished granular layer
- Focal spongiosis and acanthosis (pityriasiform spongiosis) with lymphocytic exocytosis
- Small spongiotic vesicles with lymphocytic aggregation
- Occasional dyskeratotic cells (more common in the herald patch)
- Perivascular lymphocytic infiltrate (rarely eosinophils, which then may suggest a pityriasiform drug reaction)
- Papillary dermal edema
- Red blood cell extravasation in superficial dermis and epidermis

DIFFERENTIAL DIAGNOSIS:
- **Subacute Spongiotic Dermatitis:** Cannot be distinguished from PR without clinical information.
- **Guttate Psoriasis:** Collections of neutrophils in the stratum corneum with markedly decreased granular layer.

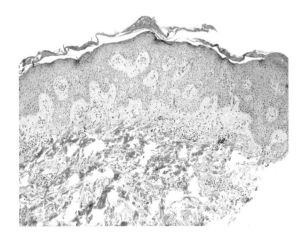

FIGURE 1-5 *Pityriasis Rosea* Epidermal hyperplasia with focal spongiosis and mounds of para-keratosis. In dermis, there are rare extravasated red blood cells with perivascular lymphocytosis.

Stasis Dermatitis

Stasis dermatitis is a common inflammatory disease that presents clinically with pruritic, erythematous scaly plaques on the lower legs. Usually it is seen in middle-aged and older patients with prior history of long-standing venous insufficiency. Ulceration may be seen as a complication in patients with long-standing stasis dermatitis.

Acroangiodermatitis is a vasoproliferative disorder that is usually seen as a complication of severe chronic venous stasis of the lower legs and the feet. Also it can be associated with paralysis of a limb, congenital arteriovenous malformation and activated protein C resistance (17, 18). Clinically, they are more commonly seen in the lower legs and feet and present as confluent, violaceous papules of the distal parts of the legs. In the majority of cases involving the legs there is concomitant stasis dermatitis.

HISTOLOGY:

▪ **Stasis Dermatitis (Figure 1-6):** Focal parakeratosis and scale crusts with mild spongiosis. In dermis, there is a dense proliferation of small blood vessels along with fibrosis, extravasated red blood cells and hemosiderin deposits. Vessels in dermis may have thick walls.

▪ **Acroangiodermatitis (Figure 1-7):** Proliferation of small blood vessels in dermis. Also, there are focal perivascular fibrosis, extravasated red blood cells and hemosiderin around the vascular proliferation. These lesions may mimic vascular neoplasms, such as Kaposi sarcoma.

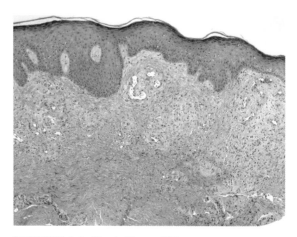

FIGURE 1-6 *Stasis Dermatitis*
The epidermis shows spongiotic changes. In dermis, there are thickened blood vessels with extravasated red blood cells and hemosiderin deposition with fibrosis.

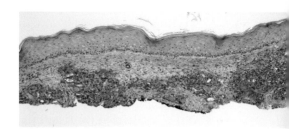

FIGURE 1-7 *Acroangiodermatitis*
The biopsy shows a clear proliferation of small vessels in dermis along with many extravasated red blood cells.

Psoriasis

Psoriasis (vulgaris) is a chronic and relapsing papulosquamous cutaneous disease characterized by erythematous skin lesions covered with silvery white scales. It commonly affects the elbow, knees, scalp, gluteal cleft, and lumbosacral area. The "Auspitz" sign can be seen in psoriasis, in which scales become headed up and abrasive removal causes small pinpoint bleeding from the small capillaries located close to the epidermis that become exposed after the abrasion. The "Koebner" phenomenon is the development of psoriasis lesions after external trauma (19). Nail involvement commonly presents as pitting of the nail plate. Approximately 10% of the cases are associated with arthritis (20).

    Guttate Psoriasis: It is often seen in children and young adults and often preceded by an upper respiratory infection (usually B-hemolytic streptococcal infection). Clinically, it is characterized by a rapid onset of small erythematous lesions, localized primarily on the trunk and proximal extremities (21).

    Generalized Pustular Psoriasis: It presents with a widespread rapid eruption of erythematous plaques (22). It may develop in three main clinical settings: 1) in patients with a long history of psoriasis of early onset (often precipitated by some external provocative agent, such as pregnancy or by the discontinuation of corticosteroids), 2) preceding psoriasis of atypical form in which the onset was late in life, and 3) pustular psoriasis, usually in patients without previous history of psoriasis.

HISTOLOGY (FIGURE 1-8A–C):
- Regular and uniform psoriasiform epidermal hyperplasia
- Confluent parakeratosis
- Neutrophilic microabscesses in stratum corneum and in epidermis (Munro and Kogoj microabscesses, respectively)
- Hypogranulosis
- Thinning of the suprapapillary plate
- Dilated capillaries in superficial dermis
- Exocytosis of lymphocytes
- Spongiosis may be seen in the early lesions and when located on the hand and feet. Erythrodermic psoriasis also may show spongiosis.
- **Guttate Psoriasis:** Characterized by mounds of parakeratosis with collection of neutrophils and focal hypogranulosis. No significant acanthosis in epidermis or dilated capillaries in superficial dermis.
- **Pustular Psoriasis:** Shows large collections of intraepidermal neutrophils. Psoriasiform hyperplasia only seen in older lesions (**Table 1-2**).
- **AIDS-associated Psoriasiform Dermatitis:** Similar histologic changes to those seen in psoriasis vulgaris but there is usually no thinning of the suprapapillary plate and there are scattered apoptotic keratinocytes within the epidermis. The papillary dermis contains plasma cells.

(continued)

Psoriasis

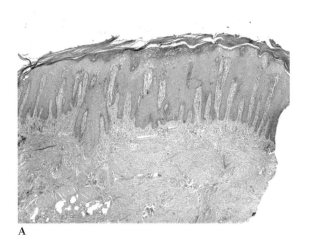

A

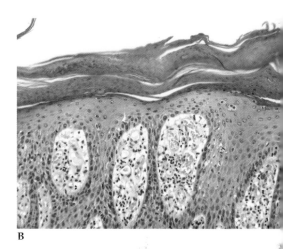

B

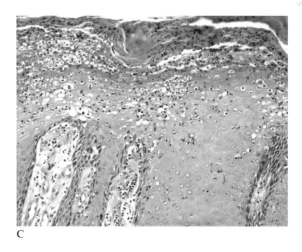

C

FIGURE 1-8 *Psoriasis*
A. Regular epidermal hyperplasia with confluent parakeratosis and increased amount of neutrophilia within both stratum corneum (Munro microabscesses) and epidermis (Kogoj microabscesses). **B.** Higher magnification showing the confluent parakeratosis, absence of granular layer, dilated capillaries in superficial dermis and thinning of suprapapillary plates. **C.** Higher magnification showing Munro and Kogoj microabscesses.

Psoriasis *(continued)*

DIFFERENTIAL DIAGNOSIS:
- Chronic Spongiotic Dermatitis: The chronic stage of eczema may look like psoriasis; however, in cases of psoriasis there are usually confluent parakeratosis and neutrophilic microabscesses. The presence of marked spongiosis (especially involving the rete ridges), retained granular layer and eosinophils will favor chronic eczema.
- Spongiotic psoriasis can be very difficult to distinguish from eczematous dermatitis; the presence of mounds of parakeratosis containing neutrophils and a subtle dermal infiltrate favor psoriasis.
- Psoriasis involving the palms and soles can be difficult to separate from eczematous dermatitis as psoriasis in these locations will show spongiosis and spongiotic microvesicles. However, the presence of multiple foci of parakeratosis with neutrophils will favor psoriasis.
- Dermatophytosis: Always perform special stains to rule out fungal microorganisms.
- Reiter disease shares many histologic features with psoriasis (see also below). However, the presence of thicker stratum corneum, spongiosis, larger neutrophilic pustules and neutrophils in dermis will slightly favor Reiter disease.

Psoriasis

TABLE 1-2 Differential Diagnosis of Subcorneal Pustules (**Figure 1-9**)

Pustular psoriasis

Acute generalized exanthematous pustulosis (AGEP)

Subcorneal pustular dermatosis

Impetigo

Fungal infections

Reiter disease

Pemphigus foliaceus

IgA pemphigus

Pustulosis palmaris et plantaris

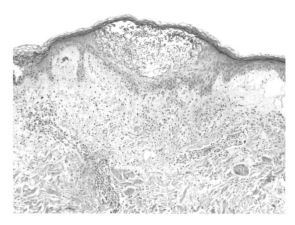

FIGURE 1-9 *Subcorneal Pustule*
There is a subcorneal blister filled with neutrophils. This particular case is an example of pustular psoriasis.

Lichen Simplex Chronicus

Lichen simplex chronicus (LSC) is characterized by thickened lichenified plaques that result from long-standing rubbing or scratching; often develops in patients with atopic dermatitis or chronic contact dermatitis. Prurigo nodularis (Picker nodule) is the same basic process but presents as circumscribed hyperkeratotic papules or nodules, usually on the extremities (23).

HISTOLOGY (FIGURE 1-10):
- ■ "Irregular" psoriasiform hyperplasia (irregular acanthosis)
- ■ Ortho/parakeratosis with wedge-shaped hypergranulosis
- ■ Vertical streaks of collagen bundles perpendicular to the epidermal surface
- ■ Mild spongiosis
- ■ Perivascular lymphocytic infiltrate

DIFFERENTIAL DIAGNOSIS:
- ■ **Prurigo Nodularis:** Typical clinical presentation is different, i.e., it usually presents as a solitary papule or nodule rather than as a plaque and shows a "crescendo" pattern of increasing epidermal hyperplasia between the periphery and the center of the lesion.

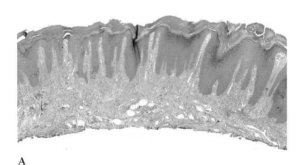
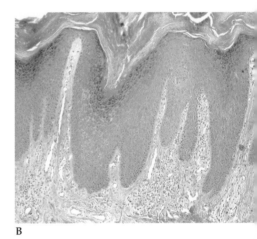

A   B

FIGURE 1-10 *Lichen Simplex Chronicus*
A. Marked compact hyperkeratosis, irregular epidermal hyperplasia, wedge-shaped hypergranulosis and fibrosis of the superficial dermis. **B.** Higher magnification shows wedge-shaped hypergranulosis and the vertical streaks of collagen bundles in dermis.

Pityriasis Rubra Pilaris

Pityriasis rubra pilaris (PRP) is a rare chronic papulosquamous disorder of unknown etiology. Clinically, it may begin as a scaling and erythematous lesion on the scalp that resembles seborrheic dermatitis. Eventually, trunk lesions coalesce into large, reddish to orange plaques with keratotic follicular papules characteristically leaving islands of spared skin. Also, palmoplantar keratoderma is characteristic and some patients may have a yellow discoloration of the nails. Lesions may progress to diffuse erythroderma (24).

HISTOLOGY (FIGURE 1-11):
- Acanthosis with short, broad rete ridges and irregular psoriasiform hyperplasia (thick suprapapillary plate)
- Mild spongiosis
- Focal or confluent hypergranulosis
- Diffuse orthokeratosis and focal parakeratosis ("checkerboard parakeratosis")
- Characteristic follicular plugs with adjacent shoulders of parakeratosis
- Mild superficial perivascular and perifollicular lymphocytic infiltrate (rare eosinophils or plasma cells)
- Focal acantholytic dyskeratosis

DIFFERENTIAL DIAGNOSIS:
- **Psoriasis:** Neutrophilic pustules, confluent parakeratosis and thinning of the suprapapillary plates are typical for psoriasis. The checkerboard pattern and follicular plugging are not seen in psoriasis.

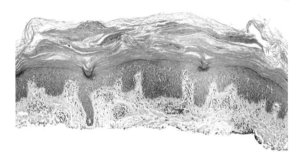

FIGURE 1-11 *Pityriasis Rubra Pilaris*
Lamellar hyperkeratosis and parakeratosis with epidermal hyperplasia and slight spongiosis.

Reiter Syndrome

Reiter syndrome is defined by arthritis, conjunctivitis, urethritis, and mucocutaneous lesions (keratoderma blennorrhagicum and balanitis circinata) (25). The peak of onset is 15-35 years of age and is much more common in males than in females. It falls under the rheumatic disease category of seronegative spondyloarthropathies. It is presumably triggered by a nongonococcal venereal disease (*Chlamydia*) or infectious diarrhea (*Shigella, Salmonella, and Yersinia*). Reiter syndrome has a genetic component as demonstrated by the association with HLA B27 (26).

HISTOLOGY (FIGURE 1-12):
Similar to pustular psoriasis:

■ Psoriasiform hyperplasia with parakeratosis
■ Spongiform pustules
■ Thinned to absent granular layer

DIFFERENTIAL DIAGNOSIS:

■ Pustular Psoriasis: The presence of thicker stratum corneum, spongiosis, larger neutrophilic pustules and neutrophils in dermis will favor Reiter disease; however, these findings may not be sufficient to separate these two entities on pure histologic grounds.
■ Other dermatoses with subcorneal pustules (see **Table 1-2**).

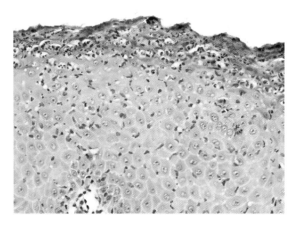

FIGURE 1-12 *Reiter Disease*
Spongiform pustules overlying the epidermal spongiosis.

Pellagra

Pellagra is a nutritional disorder secondary to niacin deficiency. Clinically, it is characterized by three "d's": dermatitis, dementia, and diarrhea (27). The cutaneous lesions are symmetrical, mostly on sun-exposed areas and areas of pressure, and present as burning erythema particularly on the dorsum of the hands and the head and neck area (28).

HISTOLOGY:
- Hyperkeratosis, parakeratosis, and acanthosis of epidermis (it may show atrophic epidermis)
- Older lesions may show psoriasiform hyperplasia
- Characteristic pallor and vacuolation of the keratinocytes in upper epidermis (granular layer)
- Pigmentation of the basal layer
- Mild lymphocytic infiltrate in superficial dermis

DIFFERENTIAL DIAGNOSIS:
- Acrodermatitis enteropathica, necrolytic migratory erythema (glucagonoma), and necrolytic acral erythema may look identical to pellagra. Thus, clinical-pathologic correlation is necessary to distinguish these entities.

Acrodermatitis Enteropathica

Acrodermatitis enteropathica is an inborn error of zinc metabolism, inherited as an autosomal recessive disorder. The acquired form is caused by inadequate dietary content of zinc (e.g., alcoholism), chronic diarrhea, and other chronic diseases that cause zinc deficiency. Clinically, the hereditary form presents in infancy and is characterized by diarrhea, dermatitis (periorificial and acral), and alopecia (29, 30).

HISTOLOGY:
- The histologic changes will depend on the stage of the lesion.
- **Early Phase:**
  - There is confluent parakeratosis above a basket-weave stratum corneum.
  - Hypergranulosis with mild spongiosis and acanthosis.
  - Pallor of the keratinocytes in upper epidermis (variable psoriasiform hyperplasia).
- **Late Phase:**
  - Psoriasiform hyperplasia with overlying parakeratosis and minimal pallor of keratinocytes.
  - Sometimes bacteria and Candida can be seen in the stratum corneum.

Necrolytic Migratory Erythema (Glucagonoma)

This dermatitis is secondary to a neoplasm, usually located in the pancreas (alpha cell tumor "glucagonoma"), which secretes excessive amounts of glucagon. Characteristic clinical findings of glucagonoma syndrome are weight loss, diabetes mellitus, anemia, and stomatitis. The skin eruption is intensely pruritic and may affect any site but most often affects the genital and anal region, the buttocks, groin, lower legs, and perioral areas (31, 32).

HISTOLOGY:
- Confluent parakeratosis
- Pallor of the keratinocytes in upper epidermis (variable psoriasiform hyperplasia)
- Abrupt necrosis of the upper layers of epidermis
- Intercellular edema of the upper Malpighian layer (clefting and acantholysis)
- Dyskeratosis and ballooning of the keratinocyte cytoplasm
- Neutrophilic infiltrate

Necrolytic Acral Erythema

This dermatosis is usually secondary to hepatitis C infection and it is limited to an acral distribution (33). Clinically, the lesions show dusky red erythematous plaques that present bilaterally on the dorsum of the feet and toes.

HISTOLOGY:
- Similar to necrolytic migratory erythema (glucagonoma) (see above)
- Parakeratosis
- Vacuolation of the mid and upper layer of epidermis
- Dyskeratosis (clue to diagnosis)

Lichenoid/Vacuolar Interface Dermatitis

2

LICHEN PLANUS

LICHENOID DRUG REACTION

BENIGN LICHENOID KERATOSIS (LICHEN PLANUS-LIKE KERATOSIS)

LICHEN NITIDUS

LICHEN STRIATUS

LICHEN SCLEROSUS (ET ATROPHICUS)

PITYRIASIS LICHENOIDES

ERYTHEMA MULTIFORME, TOXIC EPIDERMAL NECROLYSIS, AND STEVENS-JOHNSON SYNDROME

EXANTHEMATOUS/MORBILLIFORM DRUG REACTION

LUPUS ERYTHEMATOSUS
CHRONIC CUTANEOUS LUPUS
SUBACUTE CUTANEOUS LUPUS ERYTHEMATOSUS
SYSTEMIC LUPUS ERYTHEMATOSUS
NEONATAL LE

DERMATOMYOSITIS

FIXED DRUG ERUPTION

GRAFT-VERSUS-HOST DISEASE

LICHEN PLANUS

Lichen planus (LP) is clinically characterized by purple, pruritic, flat-topped papules and plaques. The lesions are most commonly seen on the flexor surfaces of the extremities, lumbar area, and glans penis. The papules may reveal a delicate white netlike pattern, referred to as Wickham striae. Lichen planus has been associated with viral infections including cases of hepatitis B and C, and HIV (34, 35).

HISTOLOGY (FIGURE 2-1A, B):
- Compact orthokeratosis
- Wedge-shaped hypergranulosis
- Irregular acanthosis (saw-toothed pattern)
- Vacuolar damage of the basal layer with many apoptotic keratinocytes (colloid bodies)
- Band-like lymphocytic infiltrate (lichenoid) mainly composed of lymphocytes and histiocytes (rare eosinophils)
- Melanophages in upper dermis (pigment incontinence)
- **Max-Joseph Spaces:** Artifactual cleft between epidermis and lichenoid infiltrate
- **Direct Immunofluorescence (DIF):** Colloid bodies in LP are positive for IgM (sometimes positive for IgA, IgG, or C3) in about 87% of the cases (**Figure 2-1C**).

VARIATIONS:
- **Hypertrophic LP:** It is usually found on the lower legs (shins) and presents as single or multiple pruritic plaques that can persist for many years. Squamous cell carcinoma may develop in long-standing lesions. Histologically, it shows prominent acanthosis and papillomatosis and minimal lichenoid inflammation along with scarring in dermis; the vacuolar damage is subtle and mainly localized to the base of the rete ridges. There may be vertical fibrosis mimicking lichen simplex chronicus. Sometimes it can be confused with squamous cell carcinoma due to the prominent epidermal hyperplasia (36, 37) (**Figure 2-2**).
- **Bullous (Vesicular) LP:** It is rare and clinically is characterized by apparent vesicles in some of the lesions. Histologically, it shows subepidermal bullae with LP-like changes (38).
- **Lichen Planus Pemphigoides:** Clinically, presents with the coexistence of LP and subepidermal blistering lesions that resemble bullous pemphigoid. Histologically, shows cell poor subepidermal bullae with only mild inflammatory response composed of lymphocytes, plasma cells and eosinophils and not much of a band-like lymphocytic infiltrate (39, 40).
- **Oral LP:** Lesions are limited to the oral cavity or can be combined with cutaneous disease. Histologically, since it occurs in a squamous mucosa (an epithelium that normally lacks granular layer) it differs from regular LP in that hypergranulosis shows just as a few cells with keratohyalin granules (41).
- **Lichen Planopilaris (LPP):** It is a type of "scarring alopecia" of the scalp. Histologically, LPP shows a dense band-like "perifollicular" lymphocytic infiltrate mainly around the infundibulum and isthmus. The interfollicular epidermis is not usually involved. In addition, there is follicular plugging and wedge-shaped hypergranulosis of the infundibulum (42, 43).

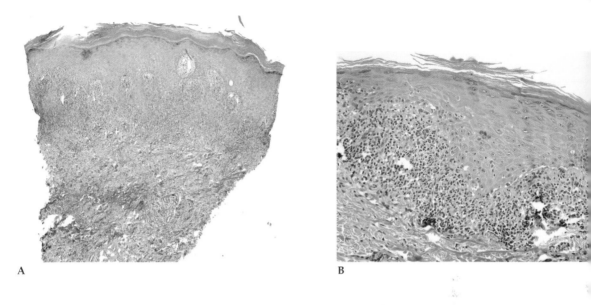

A

B

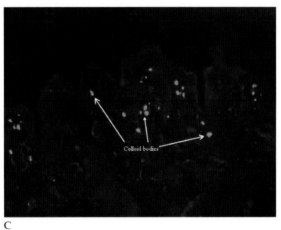

C

FIGURE 2-1 *Lichen Planus*
A. Epidermal hypergranulosis, epidermal hyperplasia, and a band-like inflammatory infiltrate in superficial dermis. **B.** Higher magnification showing the lichenoid inflammation along with basal layer vacuolization (colloid bodies) and a sawtooth pattern of the lower epidermis. **C.** Direct immunofluorescence (DIF): Colloid bodies are positive for IgM. (*Courtesy of Dr Matthew Fleming.*)

DIFFERENTIAL DIAGNOSIS:

■ **Benign Lichenoid Keratosis (BLK):** Focal parakeratosis and the presence of adjacent solar lentigo/seborrheic keratosis favor BLK. Saw-tooth hyperplasia of the epidermis is unusual in BLK. Clinically, BLK is a solitary lesion that resembles a neoplasm such as basal cell carcinoma (BCC) or squamous cell carcinoma (SCC).

■ **Lichenoid Drug Eruption:** This dermatosis may also be indistinguishable from LP. The presence of parakeratosis and absence of hypergranulosis with deeper dermal infiltrate admixed with eosinophils favor lichenoid drug eruption.

■ **Lupus Erythematosus:** Atrophy of epidermis, follicular plugging, dermal mucin, PAS-positive basement membrane, and perivascular and periadnexal dermal infiltrates with plasma cells favor lupus. DIF may be helpful by demonstrating immune complex deposition along the dermal–epidermal junction.

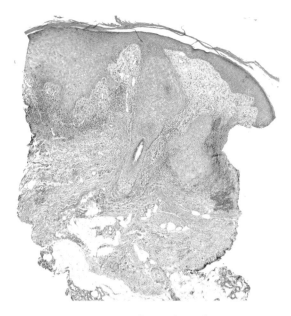

FIGURE 2-2 *Hypertrophic Lichen Planus*
Prominent irregular epidermal hyperplasia with
slight papillomatosis and mild
lichenoid inflammation.

Lichenoid drug eruptions clinically resemble LP but the lesions are often larger and without mucosal involvement. Slow resolution follows drug cessation and post-inflammatory hyperpigmentation is often pronounced. Many drugs have been involved such as beta-blockers, captopril, thiazides, and lasix (44, 45).

HISTOLOGY (FIGURE 2-3):
- ■ Parakeratosis often present
- ■ Band-like lymphocytic infiltrate
- ■ Vacuolar damage of the basal layer (colloid bodies)
- ■ Suprabasilar lymphocytosis around dyskeratotic cells
- ■ Eosinophils and plasma cells often present
- ■ In addition to the band-like infiltrate in superficial dermis, characteristically there is a deeper perivascular lymphocytic infiltrate.

DIFFERENTIAL DIAGNOSIS:
- ■ **Lichen Planus:** See above

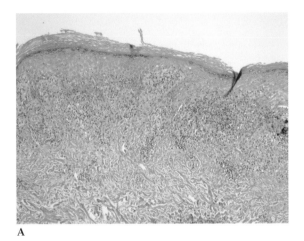 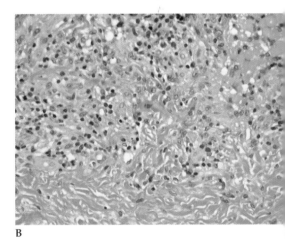

A   B

FIGURE 2-3 *Lichenoid Drug Reaction*
A. The biopsy shows a lichenoid inflammatory response that is extending to mid dermis. **B.** Higher magnification shows a mixed chronic inflammatory response admixed with many eosinophils.

BENIGN LICHENOID KERATOSIS

BLK is a frequent skin disorder that typically occurs as a single lesion on the trunk (chest), extremities and, less frequently, head and neck area of middle-aged to elderly adults. The lesion presents clinically as a tan to brown papule and is frequently clinically mistaken for basal cell carcinoma, seborrheic keratosis, or squamous cell carcinoma. BLK has been noted to involute spontaneously and may represent the inflammatory stage of regressing solar lentigines and reticulated seborrheic keratosis (46–48).

HISTOLOGY (FIGURE 2-4):
- Hyperkeratosis with partial parakeratosis
- Lichenoid pattern, in at least part of the lesion
- Vacuolar damage of the basal layer (colloid bodies)
- Hypergranulosis
- Residual "solar lentigo"/early seborrheic keratosis at the edge of the lesion (10/15% of cases)

DIFFERENTIAL DIAGNOSIS:
- **Lichen Planus:** See above
- **Lichenoid Drug Reaction:** See above

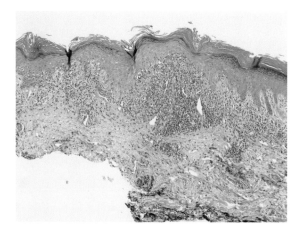

FIGURE 2-4 *Benign Lichenoid Keratosis*
Lichenoid inflammation with interface vacuolar damage of the dermal–epidermal junction.

Lichen nitidus is a rare dermatosis characterized by multiple discrete small flat-topped papules that are most commonly located on the genitalia, chest, abdomen, and arms. Children and young adult males are most commonly affected (49).

HISTOLOGY (FIGURE 2-5):

■ Nodular aggregate of mononuclear cells in the papillary dermis (lymphocytes and histiocytes)

■ Characteristic epithelioid histiocytes and multinucleated cells within the inflammatory infiltrate

■ Mild vacuolar interface damage with rare Civatte bodies

■ Overlying epidermis is atrophic and frequently covered by parakeratosis

■ Epidermis frequently shows acanthosis at the edge of the inflammatory infiltrate, creating the "ball and claw" effect

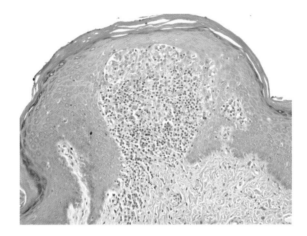

FIGURE 2-5 *Lichen Nitidus*
Nodular aggregate of histiocytes and lymphocytes in the papillary dermis creating the claw and ball effect.

LICHEN STRIATUS

Lichen striatus is a rare self-limited skin eruption that usually affects the extremities (more common left leg) and has a predilection for female children and adolescents. Clinically, presents as linear bands composed of small pink, tan, or skin-colored lichenoid papules (50–52).

HISTOLOGY (FIGURE 2-6):
■ Variable histologic picture
■ Epidermis shows mild acanthosis and spongiosis (exocytosis)
■ Superficial perivascular/lichenoid lymphohistiocytic infiltrate (rarely eosinophils)
■ Focal vacuolar interface damage of the basal layer with dyskeratotic cells
■ Characteristic inflammatory infiltrate within reticular dermis and extending around the eccrine glands
■ Some cases may show Langerhans cell microabscesses in epidermis

DIFFERENTIAL DIAGNOSIS:
■ Other lichenoid dermatosis such as lichen planus and lichen nitidus may show similar features. The presence of spongiosis and inflammatory infiltrate around the eccrine structures are not characteristic features of lichen planus. In lichen nitidus, the inflammatory infiltrate is confined to widened dermal papillae and has more histiocytic infiltrate with occasional multinucleated giant cells.

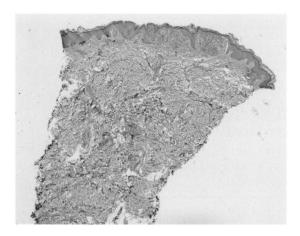

FIGURE 2-6 *Lichen Striatus*
Subtle lichenoid inflammation in dermis. Note the inflammatory response around eccrine ducts.

LICHEN SCLEROSUS (ET ATROPHICUS)

Lichen sclerosus (LS) most commonly occurs in the anogenital region of middle aged and elderly women. Clinically, LS starts as ivory to white papules evolving to erythematous macules and plaques that resolve as an atrophic patch with a characteristic "cigarette-paper" appearance. Extragenital lesions can also be seen in trunk, neck, and upper and lower extremities. Lesions involving the penis are designated balanitis xerotica obliterans (BXO) (53–55).

HISTOLOGY (FIGURE 2-7):
- Hyperkeratosis with follicular plugging
- Atrophy of the epidermis
- Mild interface vacuolar damage
- Marked edema and homogenization of the collagen in upper dermis
- **Note:** Early lesions show a characteristic lichenoid infiltrate simulating LP

DIFFERENTIAL DIAGNOSIS:
- Early lesions of LS can resemble lichen planus; however, clinically they have different presentations and LS can show focal subepidermal edema.
- Morphea may be similar to the late stage of lichen sclerosus, so called LS/morphea overlap. However, the epidermis in morphea can be atrophic but does not show the hydropic degeneration of the basal layer or the follicular plugging characteristic of LS. Also, in morphea there is no homogenization of the superficial dermis as it contains elastic fibers.

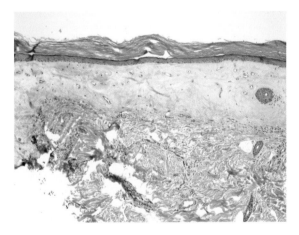

FIGURE 2-7 *Lichen Sclerosus (et Atrophicus)* Hyperkeratosis, atrophy of epidermis and marked edema and homogenization of the collagen in upper dermis.

Pityriasis lichenoides is the term given to a group of rare cutaneous disorders ranging from acute ulceronecrotic lesions that rapidly evolve, called pityriasis lichenoides et varioliformis acuta (Mucha-Habermann disease), to small, scaling, benign-appearing more chronic papules called pityriasis lichenoides chronica (PLC) (56–58).

Pityriasis lichenoides et varioliformis acuta (PLEVA) (Figure 2-8A–C)

- Corneal layer with parakeratosis and scaly crust with neutrophils
- Dense perivascular lymphocytic infiltrate in papillary dermis extending into the reticular dermis (sometimes in a wedge-shaped pattern)
- Marked interface vacuolar damage of the DEJ (sometimes vesiculation)
- Cohesive collection of Langerhans cell in the upper layers of epidermis
- Lymphocytic exocytosis and dyskeratotic keratinocytes
- Red cell extravasation in superficial dermis and epidermis
- Focal epidermal necrosis
- Rarely lymphocytes display hyperchromatic, convoluted nuclei
- **IHC:** Mostly CD3 with a predominance of CD8+ T cells
- Lymphocytes are mostly CD3+

Pityriasis Lichenoides Et Varioliformis Acuta (PLEVA)

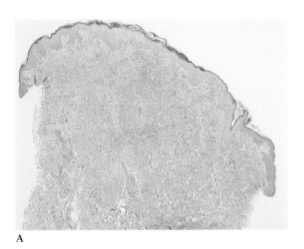

A

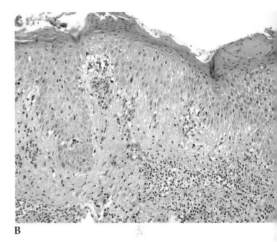

B

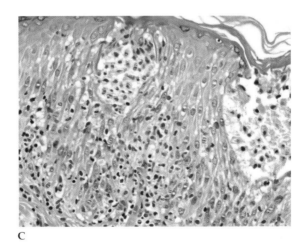

C

FIGURE 2-8 *Pityriasis Lichenoides Et Varioliformis Acuta (PLEVA)*
A. Wedge-shaped inflammatory infiltrate in dermis with interface damage. **B.** Higher magnification showing the interface vacuolar damage, extravasated red blood cells and lymphocytic exocytosis. **C.** Higher magnification showing the characteristic Langerhans cell microabscesses within the epidermis.

Pityriasis Lichenoides Chronica (PLC) (Figure 2-9)

HISTOLOGY:
- Confluent parakeratosis
- Lesser degree of superficial perivascular and lichenoid lymphocytic infiltrate
- Interface vacuolar damage
- Mild epidermal spongiosis and acanthosis
- Rare dyskeratotic keratinocytes
- Red cell extravasation in superficial dermis
- **IHC:** Mostly CD3 with a slight predominance of CD4 over CD8 + T cells

DIFFERENTIAL DIAGNOSIS:
- PLEVA might be confused histologically with arthropod bite, subacute eczema, or mycosis fungoides. By immunohistochemistry the inflammatory infiltrate in PLEVA is CD3, CD8, and CD7 +, rarely lacking CD2 and CD5 expression. PLEVA can show monoclonality by TCR studies. Furthermore, some patients with PLEVA have been shown to progress to frank mycosis fungoides (59).

Pityriasis Lichenoides Chronica (PLC)

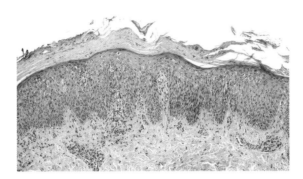

FIGURE 2-9 *Pityriasis Lichenoides Chronica* Mild interface vacuolar damage with lymphocytic exocytosis and mild perivascular lymphocytic infiltrate in dermis.

ERYTHEMA MULTIFORME, TOXIC EPIDERMAL NECROLYSIS, STEVENS-JOHNSON SYNDROME

There are some controversies regarding the definition of erythema multiforme (EM), toxic epidermal necrolysis (TEN), and Stevens-Johnson Syndrome (SJS). EM is a self-limited condition characterized by symmetrically distributed maculopapular targetoid lesions, most often on the hands, feet, elbows, or knees but may involve almost any area. SJS presents with flat atypical targetoid lesions, some of them with necrosis, and epidermal detachment in < 10% of the body surface area. Some authorities consider TEN to represent an extreme form of EM, as characterized by widespread erythema, extensive blistering, and erosions and by epidermal necrosis involving > 30% of the body surface. EM is frequently associated with infection; the most common offending organisms are herpes simplex viruses (Type I and II) and Mycoplasma, although other causes include viral, fungal, and bacterial infections. Medications, most commonly sulfonamides, are also associated with EM. Also, recurrent cases of EM have been associated with increased incidence of HLA-B15, HLA-DR53, and HLA-B35; patients with mucosal involvement have been associated with HLA-DQB1*0302 and HLA-DQB1*0402 (60–62).

HISTOLOGY (FIGURE 2-10A):
- Prototype of interface dermatitis (hydropic changes and dyskeratosis)
- Satellite cell necrosis (individual keratinocytes surrounded by lymphocytes)
- Lymphocytic infiltrate around the superficial vascular plexuses and along the DEJ
- In well-developed lesions, extensive vacuolar degeneration leads to subepidermal clefting or vesiculation
- Eosinophils occasionally (when numerous they will favor drug-induced EM)
- **TEN/SJS:** Full-thickness epidermal necrosis with subepidermal bullae associated with sparser interface dermatitis and with frequent involvement of the sweat duct epithelium (**Figure 2-10B**)

DIFFERENTIAL DIAGNOSIS:
- Fixed drug eruption (shows more melanophages in superficial dermis)
- Viral exanthem
- GVHD
- Phototoxic dermatitis
- Connective tissue disease (lupus, dermatomyositis, etc.)

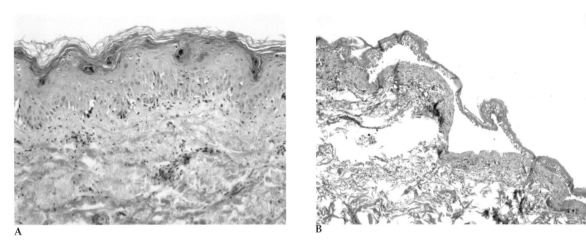

FIGURE 2-10 A. Erythema multiforme. Interface dermatitis with hydropic changes and dyskeratotic keratinocytes along satellite-cell necrosis. **B.** Toxic epidermal necrolysis. Note the subepidermal bullae with confluent necrosis of the overlying epidermis.

EXANTHEMATOUS/MORBILLIFORM DRUG REACTION

This entity accounts for the most common form of cutaneous drug eruption. Clinically, it is characterized by salmon-colored macular or papular lesions often arranged in a gyrate or reticular pattern. The lesions are noted most commonly within 1–2 weeks after starting the drug, and they clear within 1–6 weeks after withdrawal. Implicated agents include penicillin, ampicillin, sulfonamides, amoxicillin, isoniazide, etc. (63, 64).

HISTOLOGY (FIGURE 2-11):
■ Subtle interface dermatitis with dyskeratotic cells
■ Minimal epidermal changes (spongiosis, exocytosis)
■ Superficial perivascular lymphohistiocytic infiltrate with rare eosinophils

DIFFERENTIAL DIAGNOSIS:
■ Graft Versus Host Disease (GVHD): Presence of numerous eosinophils may favor a drug reaction; however, cases of GVHD may show a focal eosinophilic infiltrate.
■ Erythema multiforme
■ Fixed drug eruption

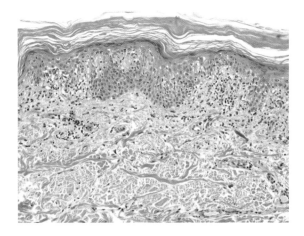

FIGURE 2-11 *Exanthematous/Morbilliform Drug Reaction*
Mild interface vacuolar damage with spongiosis and acanthosis. Also, superficial perivascular lymphocytic infiltrate with eosinophils.

Lupus erythematosus (LE) is an autoimmune disorder that affects multiple organ systems and is associated with antibodies directed against cell nuclei. Cutaneous forms of LE present in several clinical forms and they are more common than systemic lupus. Cutaneous disease is the presenting symptom in 23% to 28% of cases of systemic lupus patients, and 75% to 88% of SLE patients manifest with at least one cutaneous symptom. Cutaneous changes in LE may be subdivided according to the clinical presentation or its duration (acute, subacute, or chronic). Some authors consider that the clinical variants of lupus cannot be separated on the basis of histology alone (65, 66).

Chronic Cutaneous Lupus

Discoid lupus erythematosus (DLE) is the most common subtype and presents clinically with erythematous plaques of varying sizes associated with scaling. In the disseminated form of DLE, SLE may eventually develop in up to 20% of these patients (67, 68).

Tumid lupus is the dermal form of LE without surface or epidermal changes. Clinically, it presents with indurated plaques and nodules without erythema (69, 70).

Lupus Profundus/Lupus Panniculitis: Clinically, presents with deep-seated nodules involving subcutaneous tissue; most commonly on the trunk. Up to 2/3 of affected patients have DLE (see panniculitis section).

Subacute Cutaneous Lupus Erythematosus

Subacute cutaneous lupus erythematosus (SCLE) represents approximately 10% of all cases of LE, and is characterized clinically by widespread nonscarring annular erythematous scaly lesions. Approximately 50% of patients with SCLE have manifestations of systemic disease. SCLE may occur not only in patients with SLE, but can also be associated with patients with Sjögren syndrome, rheumatoid arthritis, medications (drug-induced SCLE), and in patients with malignant neoplasms treated with radiotherapy (71–73).

Systemic Lupus Erythematosus

Systemic lupus erythematosus (SLE) is a complex disease with myriad manifestations. In addition to cutaneous disease, patients frequently manifest immunologic, hematologic, neurologic, and renal disorders as well as serositis, arthritis, and oral ulcers. Cutaneous manifestations occur in 75%–88% of patients, the most characteristic being the malar "butterfly" rash. Patients with SLE may also develop DLE and SCLE (74).

Neonatal LE

It is a rare condition that occurs in infants born to mothers with anti-Ro (SS-A) or anti-La (SS-B) autoantibodies. The mothers of affected infants frequently do not have clinical manifestations of connective tissue disease; however, they may develop other manifestations, particularly Sjögren syndrome or leukocytoclastic vasculitis. Most important, infants with neonatal lupus erythematosus may develop cardiac manifestations, usually congenital heart block. Clinically the lesions can result in SCLE-like eruptions showing annular scaly plaques (75, 76).

HISTOLOGY (FIGURE 2-12A–C):
- Interface dermatitis with vacuolization and dyskeratosis (sometimes colloid bodies can be observed in the papillary dermis)
- Usually epidermal atrophy (epidermis can be hyperplastic)
- Follicular plugging and corneal hyperkeratosis (especially in discoid lupus)
- Thickened basement membrane (PAS +)
- Increased mucin in dermis (colloidal iron or Alcian blue +)
- Perivascular, periadnexal infiltrate of lymphocytes and plasma cells (sometimes it can be lichenoid)
- No eosinophils (except for bullous LE)
- **Bullous LE:** Variant of SLE; it shows a subepidermal blister usually with many neutrophils and scattered eosinophils but it can show only mononuclear cells. When neutrophils predominate the differential diagnosis includes dermatitis herpetiformis and linear IgA.
- **Tumid Lupus:** Shows a perivascular and periappendiceal mononuclear cell infiltrate and dermal mucin deposition and minimal to no epidermal changes (**Figure 2-12D**).

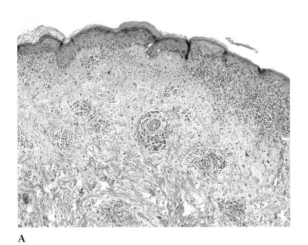

A

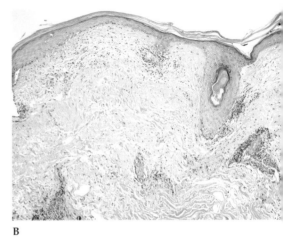

B

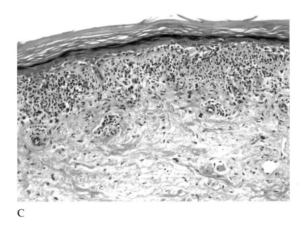

C

FIGURE 2-12 *Lupus Erythematosus*
A. Interface vacuolar damage with perifollicular and perivascular lymphocytic infiltrate. **B.** Mild interface vacuolar damage with mucin deposition in dermis along with perifollicular and perivascular lymphocytic infiltrate. **C.** Hyperkeratosis with epidermal atrophy and interface vacuolar damage of the dermal–epidermal junction.

DIRECT IMMUNOFLUORESCENCE (DIF) IN LE (LUPUS BAND TEST):

- Lesional skin in patients with LE usually demonstrates a combination of immuno-globulins (IgG, IgA, and IgM) and complement (C3) at the basement membrane in a granular pattern along the DEJ (**Figure 2-13**).
- IgM is most commonly identified and IgG appears to be the most specific for LE.
- The lupus band test is seen in 60% of patients with SCLE, 50% of infants with neonatal lupus, 50%–94% of patients with SLE and 60%–80% of patients with DLE.
- When the lupus band test is performed on non-lesional skin, a positive result indicates SLE.
- In general a positive lupus band test on non-lesional skin does not occur in the setting of DLE or SCLE.

DIFFERENTIAL DIAGNOSIS:

- Dermatomyositis
- Lichen sclerosus
- Atrophic lichen planus

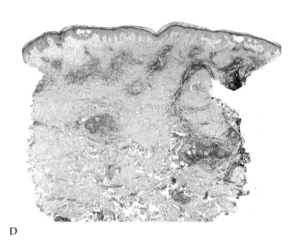

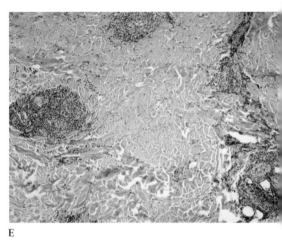

D

E

FIGURE 2-12 *Tumid Lupus Erythematosus*
D. Superficial and mid dermal perivascular lymphocytic infiltrate without interface vacuolar damage in epidermis. **E.** Higher magnification showing the dense perivascular lymphocytic infiltrate with dermal mucin deposition.

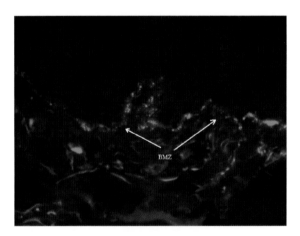

FIGURE 2-13 *Lupus Erythematosus*
Direct immunofluorescence (DIF): C3 in basement membrane with a granular pattern along the dermal–epidermal junction. (*Courtesy of Dr Matthew Fleming.*)

DERMATOMYOSITIS

Dermatomyositis (DM) is a connective tissue disease usually characterized by myositis and dermatitis. Skin manifestations are quite distinctive and include erythematous papules and plaques, periungual erythema, erythematous papules on the skin overlying the metacarpophalangeal joints (Gottron papules) and characteristic reddish, purple periorbital swelling (heliotrope flower rash). There are commonly periungual telangiectasias and a characteristic cuticular change with hypertrophy of the cuticle and small, hemorrhagic infarcts. Importantly, in adults, dermatomyositis may be associated with internal malignancy in 30% of patients. Association with pulmonary interstitial fibrosis can be seen in patients with DM and an important indicator is the presence of anti-Jo-1 antibody (77–79).

HISTOLOGY (FIGURE 2-14):
- Usually atrophic epidermis (it can be normal)
- Subtle interface dermatitis with scattered lymphocytes
- Thickened basement membrane (PAS +)
- Dermal mucin and edema
- Sparse lymphocytic infiltrate in superficial vessels
- Superficial vessels show vascular drop out with endothelial cell necrosis and degeneration
- DIF is negative but there is C5b-9 complex deposition in the superficial dermal blood vessels walls

DIFFERENTIAL DIAGNOSIS:
- **LE:** The main distinction of DM with LE is that LE shows mostly a deep inflammatory infiltrate and prominent deep dermal mucin deposition, whereas in DM both features are limited to the superficial dermis.

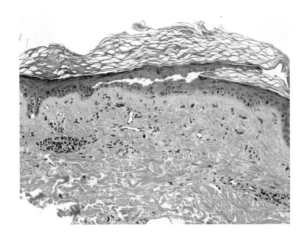

FIGURE 2-14 *Dermatomyositis* Atrophic epidermis with subtle interface damage and degeneration of the basement membrane.

Fixed drug eruption (FDE) is characterized by one or more well-defined, erythematous, dusky, purple to brown patches or plaques showing predilection for the extremities and external genitalia. The main clinical feature is the recurrence in the same location after re-ingestion of the offending medication. The implicated drugs include tetracycline, barbiturates, phenolphthalein, sulfonamides, and non-steroidal anti-inflammatory agents (80, 81).

HISTOLOGY (FIGURE 2-15):
- Interface dermatitis with dyskeratosis
- Superficial and deep perivascular infiltrate composed of lymphocytes, histiocytes, neutrophils, and eosinophils
- Subepidermal vesiculation occasionally
- A characteristic feature is the presence of prominent dermal melanophages in the upper dermis reflecting prior epidermal damage (recurrent process)

DIFFERENTIAL DIAGNOSIS:
- **EM:** FDE shows a superficial and deep, heavier inflammatory infiltrate that often contains neutrophils and eosinophils. Furthermore, the presence of melanophages aids in the differential diagnosis. Clinical correlation is of paramount importance.

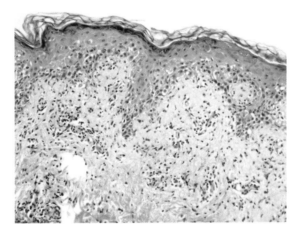

FIGURE 2-15 *Fixed Drug Eruption*
Interface dermatitis with many dyskeratotic cells. Note the melanophages and rare eosinophils in superficial dermis.

GRAFT-VERSUS-HOST DISEASE

Graft-versus-host disease (GVHD) is a multisystemic disorder that occurs in immuno-compromised patients who receive functional T-lymphocytes. Up to 70% of patients receiving allogeneic bone marrow transplants develop GVHD, and less frequently GVHD may develop after transfusion of non-irradiated blood products or transplantation of solid tissue. Clinically, GVHD shows a macular eruption, starting on the trunk and then extending to the extremities. Severe cases may be associated with bullae and extensive desquamation. GVHD is usually subdivided arbitrarily into two groups: acute GVHD occurring within the first 100 days following transplantation and chronic GVHD presenting after that period. We recommend not making a definitive diagnosis of acute GVHD unless the biopsy is taken at least 14 days after BMT (to avoid confusion with chemotherapy effect and engrafting, since the latter two entities can be very similar to GVHD) (82–84).

HISTOLOGY (FIGURE 2-16):
- **Acute Phase:** Characterized by interface dermatitis with minimal to moderate lymphocytic infiltration along the DEJ. The presence of dyskeratotic cells with satellite lymphocytosis is characteristic. Occasional subepidermal blister.
- **Chronic Phase:** It usually starts with focal hyperkeratosis and hypergranulosis. Later lesions may show lichenoid dermatitis resembling lichen planus or prominent sclerosis and hyalinization resembling lichen sclerosus or morphea/scleroderma.
- A characteristic feature of GVHD is that it involves the hair follicle and the acrosyringium as shown by the presence of necrotic keratinocytes in those adnexal structures.

DIFFERENTIAL DIAGNOSIS:
- Other dermatosis with interface dermatitis such as EM, drug reactions, viral infections, etc. The presence of eosinophils is not a real discriminator between acute GVHD and drug reactions. In our experience, GVHD has a relatively high number of necrotic keratinocytes in relation to the sparse lymphocytic infiltrate. In contrast, drug reactions have relatively dense lymphocytic infiltrate and usually only scattered necrotic keratinocytes. Clinical history is of critical value.

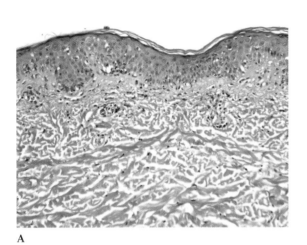 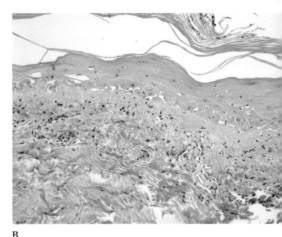

A   B

FIGURE 2-16 *Graft-Versus-Host Disease*
A. Interface dermatitis with mild lymphocytic infiltration along the dermal–epidermal junction. There are many dyskeratotic cells. **B.** Higher magnification shows a marked interface vacuolar damage with large apoptotic keratinocytes.

Bullous and Acantholytic Dermatoses

3

INTRAEPIDERMAL CLEFTING
PEMPHIGUS VULGARIS

PEMPHIGUS FOLIACEUS/FOGO SELVAGEM/PEMPHIGUS
  ERYTHEMATOSUS

PARANEOPLASTIC PEMPHIGUS

PEMPHIGUS VEGETANS

IGA PEMPHIGUS

HAILEY-HAILEY DISEASE (BENIGN FAMILIAL PEMPHIGUS)

DARIER DISEASE (KERATOSIS FOLLICULARIS)

GROVER DISEASE (TRANSIENT ACANTHOLYTIC DERMATOSIS)

ACROPUSTULOSIS OF INFANCY

TRANSIENT NEONATAL PUSTULAR MELANOSIS

ERYTHEMA TOXICUM NEONATARUM

SUBEPIDERMAL CLEFTING
BULLOUS PEMPHIGOID

CICATRICIAL PEMPHIGOID

PEMPHIGOID GESTATIONIS (HERPES GESTATIONIS)

DERMATITIS HERPETIFORMIS

LINEAR IGA DERMATOSIS

BULLOUS LUPUS ERYTHEMATOSUS

PORPHYRIA CUTANEA TARDA

EPIDERMOLYSIS BULLOSA

EPIDERMOLYSIS BULLOSA ACQUISITA

Pemphigus Vulgaris

Pemphigus vulgaris (PV) is an autoimmune blistering disease affecting the skin and mucous membranes that is mediated by circulating autoantibodies directed against keratinocyte cell surfaces. PV antibody binds to keratinocyte cell surface molecules and desmoglein 3 (130 kD), triggering a cellular process that results in acantholysis. PV is most commonly seen in middle-aged and elderly adults although rarely children may be affected. Widespread vesicles, bullae, and erosions involve the oral mucosa, face, scalp, central chest, and intertriginous areas. Oral mucosal involvement is frequently the first manifestation of disease. Drugs, most commonly penicillamine and captopril, may be associated with a pemphigus-like eruption (85–90).

HISTOLOGY (FIGURE 3-1):
- Intraepidermal vesicle with cleavage above the basal cell layer of epidermis (intact single cell layer of basal cells referred to as "tombstones").
- Variable inflammatory infiltrate within the vesicle (lymphocytes, eosinophils).
- The suprabasal vesicle extends into the epithelium of the adnexa.
- The dermis shows a variable superficial perivascular mixed inflammatory infiltrate, including lymphocytes and occasional eosinophils.
- **Drug-induced PV:** The blister may show a cleavage plane near the granular cell layer (similar to pemphigus foliaceus, see below) or in the suprabasal plane (thus similar to PV).
- **Direct immunofluorescence (DIF):** Reveals a characteristic deposit of IgG (IgG1 and IgG4) and sometimes C3 in a "lacelike" pattern outlining the intercellular zones of epithelial keratinocytes (**Figure 3-2**).

DIFFERENTIAL DIAGNOSIS:
- Other dermatoses with intraepidermal vesicles such as Hailey-Hailey disease and Grover disease. In the latter diseases there is no involvement of skin adnexa and immunofluorescence studies are negative.

Pemphigus Vulgaris

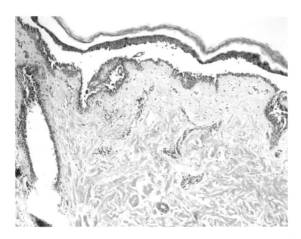

FIGURE 3-1 *Pemphigus Vulgaris*
Suprabasilar cleft in a "tombstone" pattern.

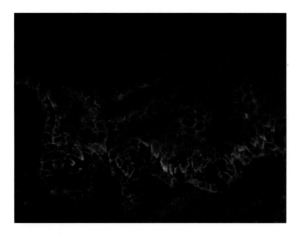

FIGURE 3-2 *Pemphigus Vulgaris*
Direct immunofluorescence (DIF):
Characteristic deposit of IgG in a "lacelike"
pattern outlining the intercellular zones of
epithelial keratinocytes. (*Courtesy of Dr Matthew
Fleming.*)

Pemphigus Foliaceus/Fogo Selvagem/ Pemphigus Erythematosus

Pemphigus foliaceus (PF) is a rare form of pemphigus, with a more benign course, seen in adults and characterized by widespread patches and fragile blisters, erosions, and scale crust. The blisters in PF are induced by IgG (IgG4 subclass) autoantibodies directed against a cell adhesion molecule, desmoglein 1 (160 kD), located mainly in the granular layer of the epidermis. Fogo selvagem or endemic PF is an endemic disease in the rivers of Brazil. It is clinically, pathophysiologically, and histologically similar to PF and it may be mediated by an arthropod vector (*Simulium* species). Pemphigus erythematosus (PE) (Senear-Usher syndrome) is characterized by an erythematous rash of the central face that resembles the butterfly rash of lupus erythematosus. Rarely can it be associated with thymoma. The target antigen of PE is desmoglein 1, as seen in PF and fogo selvagem (91–93).

HISTOLOGY (FIGURE 3-3):
- PF, PE, and fogo selvagem are characterized by superficial vesicle formation with the plane of cleavage located within subcorneal keratinocytes near the level of the granular cell layer or beneath the stratum corneum.
- Eosinophilic spongiosis can be apparent.
- **DIF:** PF, PE, and fogo selvagem show labeling of the intercellular region of the epidermis for IgG with possible accentuation in superficial epidermis. In PE, DIF also shows a linear or granular IgG (sometimes also C3) at the epidermal basement membrane.
- **Note:** Sometimes the roof of the fragile blister is not observed, having peeled off during the biopsy procedure or during processing. The biopsy then may show dyskeratotic cells on the surface of the epidermis and lack granular cell layer and stratum corneum.

DIFFERENTIAL DIAGNOSIS:
- **Impetigo:** This superficial bacterial infection may be associated with a subcorneal vesicle containing numerous neutrophils and rare acantholytic keratinocytes.

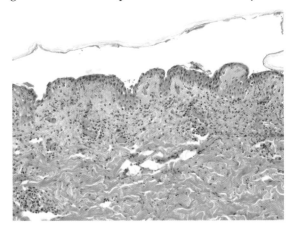

FIGURE 3-3 *Pemphigus Foliaceus*
Superficial blister with the plane of cleavage located within subcorneal layer.

Paraneoplastic Pemphigus

Paraneoplastic pemphigus (PP) is a severely debilitating blistering disease affecting skin and mucous membranes in patients with some types of malignancies. The most common are hematopoietic, particularly chronic lymphocytic leukemia. Clinically, the lesions in PP are variable and may show bullae, lichenoid or erythema multiforme-like lesions along with painful oral ulcerations. In PP, the antibodies target epithelial proteins in desmosomes and hemidesmosomes, including desmoplakins 1 and 2, desmoglein 1 and 3, BP Ag 1, envoplakin, plectin, and periplakin (94, 95).

HISTOLOGY (FIGURE 3-4):

- ▪ PP shows a combination of a vacuolar interface dermatitis resembling erythema multiforme, lichenoid reaction similar to lichen planus as well as suprabasal acantholysis resembling PV.
- ▪ **DIF:** Reveals intercellular labeling with IgG throughout the whole thickness of the epidermis, whereas C3 is only seen on the lower epidermis. Also, there is labeling of the epidermal basement membrane with IgG and C3 in a granular or linear pattern.

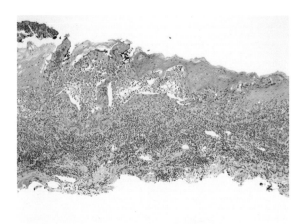

FIGURE 3-4 *Paraneoplastic Pemphigus*
Combination of vacuolar interface dermatitis with lichenoid inflammation. Minimal suprabasilar acantholysis.

Pemphigus Vegetans

Pemphigus vegetans is a rare variant of pemphigus that affects the intertriginous areas, such as axilla and groin. Two variants of pemphigus vegetans have been described. The Neumann type initially shows clinical lesions similar to pemphigus vulgaris but the lesions eventually progress into vegetating plaques. The Hallopeau type starts as pustular erosion and usually shows a relatively benign clinical course (96).

HISTOLOGY (FIGURE 3-5):
- Pseudoepitheliomatous hyperplasia
- Intraepidermal clefts (mainly suprabasal)
- Intraepidermal pustules composed mainly of neutrophils and eosinophils
- **DIF:** Squamous intercellular IgG

DIFFERENTIAL DIAGNOSIS:
- **Pyoderma Vegetans:** Associated with inflammatory bowel disease (mainly ulcerative colitis). DIF is negative.
- Halogenoderma.

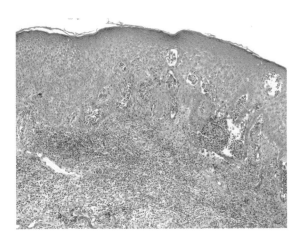

FIGURE 3-5 *Pemphigus Vegetans*
Epidermal hyperplasia with focal intraepidermal clefting and many pustules with neutrophils and eosinophils.

IgA Pemphigus

IgA Pemphigus is a rare dermatosis primarily seen in middle-aged and elderly individuals. Clinically, it presents with flaccid pustules in an annular arrangement; it usually affects the axilla and groin. Two types have been described: the subcorneal pustular dermatosis (SPD) type (desmocollin 1) and the intraepidermal neutrophilic (IEN) dermatosis type (desmoglein 1 or desmoglein 3 in a subset of patients) (97, 98).

HISTOLOGY:
- **SPD Type:** Subcorneal vesiculopustules with focal acanthosis
- **IEN Type:** Intraepidermal vesiculopustules with neutrophils
- **DIF:** IgA deposition in the intercellular epidermis with intensity in the upper layers especially in the SPD type

DIFFERENTIAL DIAGNOSIS:
The SPD variant may look like Sneddon-Wilkinson syndrome, pustular psoriasis, acute generalized exanthematous pustulosis (AGEP), Reiter disease, pustular impetigo, etc. DIF will be very helpful in this differential diagnosis.

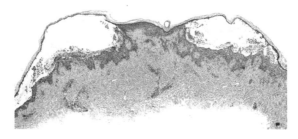

FIGURE 3-6 *IgA Pemphigus*
The biopsy shows multiple large subcorneal pustules. They are filled predominantly with neutrophils, but a few eosinophils and acantholytic keratinocytes are observed.

Hailey-Hailey Disease
(Benign Familial Pemphigus)

Hailey-Hailey disease is a rare acantholytic, autosomal, dominantly inherited genodermatosis. Hailey-Hailey disease, which most commonly presents in young adulthood, is characterized by grouped flaccid vesicles and erosions that most commonly involve the intertriginous regions. Hailey-Hailey disease probably results from a genetic defect in a calcium pump protein with multiple mutations in *ATP2C1*, a gene localized on chromosome 3q21-24 (99–101).

HISTOLOGY (FIGURE 3-7):
- Characteristic incomplete acantholysis giving a "dilapidated brick wall" appearance.
- Sometimes there are dyskeratotic cells thus resembling Darier and Grover disease.
- Early lesions occasionally show a vesicle with a suprabasal cleft thus mimicking pemphigus vulgaris.
- Adnexal structures are spared.
- **DIF:** Negative

DIFFERENTIAL DIAGNOSIS:
- **PV, Darier Disease, Grover Disease:** Hailey-Hailey disease characteristically spares follicular epithelium.

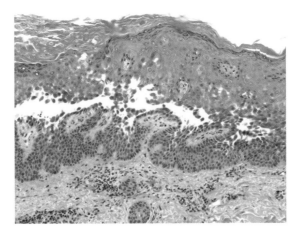

FIGURE 3-7 *Hailey-Hailey Disease*
Incomplete epidermal acantholysis in a "dilapidated brick wall" pattern.

Darier Disease
(Keratosis Follicularis)

Darier disease is a rare autosomal dominantly inherited genodermatosis characterized by symmetric widespread, keratotic yellow-brown papules and plaques that tend to involve the chest, back, neck, ears, forehead, and scalp; it presents most commonly during the first and second decades of life. Almost all patients show subtle acral changes, particularly alternating white and red streaks on the fingernails with notches at the free margin. Some patients have mutations in the ATP2A2 (12q23-q24) gene (102–104).

HISTOLOGY (FIGURE 3-8):
■ Characteristically it shows acantholysis, dyskeratosis, and overlying parakeratosis.
■ Characteristic corps ronds, which are squamous cells in the granular cell layer with abundant keratohyaline granules and pyknotic nucleus surrounded by a halo and corps grains which are located in the horny layer and represent flattened round cells with cigar-shaped nuclei.
■ An orthokeratotic plug with parakeratosis often overlies the lesion.
■ **DIF:** Negative

DIFFERENTIAL DIAGNOSIS:
■ **PV:** Suprabasal cleft formation mimics PV; however, the accompanying extensive dyskeratosis would be unusual in the latter.
■ Grover disease

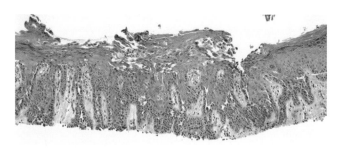

FIGURE 3-8 *Darier Disease*
Acantholysis, dyskeratosis, and overlying parakeratosis with characteristic corp grain and corp ronds. Note the orthokeratotic plug with parakeratosis overlaying the lesion.

Grover Disease
(Transient Acantholytic Dermatosis)

Grover disease is an acquired disease predominantly seen in middle-aged and elderly men. It is characterized by polymorphic erythematous papules that tend to involve the trunk, chest, and, less frequently, extremities. Since the lesions frequently occur after sun exposure, sweating, radiation, and drug ingestion, it has been proposed that Grover disease is related to alteration of sweat gland secretion (105, 106). A related entity is Galli-Galli disease, in which the clinical presentation is identical to Dowling-Degos disease (hyperpigmented macules in a reticulate or widespread distribution), but histologically shows suprabasal non-dyskeratotic acantholysis.

HISTOLOGY (FIGURE 3-9A, B):
- Several histological patterns have been observed in Grover disease:
  - Spongiosis, parakeratosis, and dyskeratosis resembling Darier disease (most common pattern)
  - Acantholysis resembling Hailey-Hailey disease or pemphigus vulgaris
  - Spongiosis with few acantholytic cells resembling spongiotic dermatitis
- Superficial perivascular lymphocytic infiltrate including eosinophils
- **DIF:** Negative

DIFFERENTIAL DIAGNOSIS:
- Grover disease lesions tend to exhibit discrete foci with multiple patterns in the same biopsy (e.g., spongiosis, acantholysis, and dyskeratosis). One pattern may predominate but more than one of these histological patterns may be present. The presence of eosinophils will favor the diagnosis of Grover disease over Darier disease.

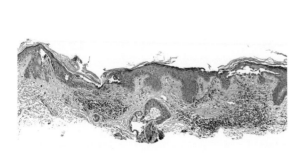
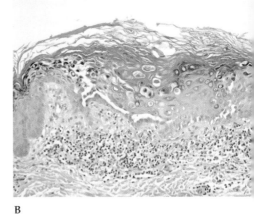

A   B

FIGURE 3-9 *Grover Disease*
Focal parakeratosis, acantholysis, and dyskeratosis.

Acropustulosis of Infancy

Acropustulosis of infancy presents with intensely pruritic vesicles or pustules that are 1 to 3 mm in diameter most commonly located on the palms and soles. It usually presents at birth or during the first year of life. Lesions tend to heal with hyperpigmentation and resolve by 2 years of age. Some cases have been reported to be associated with atopic dermatitis (108, 109).

HISTOLOGY:
- Intraepidermal or subcorneal pustules with neutrophils and eosinophils
- Mild papillary edema
- Superficial perivascular mixed inflammatory infiltrate

DIFFERENTIAL DIAGNOSIS:
- Transient Neonatal Pustular Melanosis: Identical to acropustulosis of infancy; clinical data are necessary for the distinction.
- Impetigo, subcorneal pustular dermatosis and dermatophytosis may look alike.

Transient Neonatal Pustular Melanosis

Transient neonatal pustular melanosis (TNPM) presents clinically as flaccid vesico-pustules with a predilection for the face, trunk, and genital area. It usually presents at birth. Some experts believe that erythema toxicum neonatarum represents the same disease in different phases (110, 111).

HISTOLOGY:
- Intracorneal and subcorneal pustules with neutrophils and eosinophils
- Derma inflammation (neutrophils, lymphocytes, and eosinophils)

DIFFERENTIAL DIAGNOSIS:
- Acropustulosis of infancy

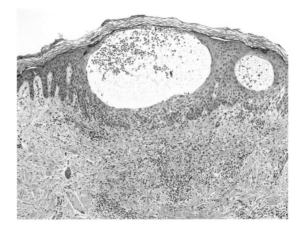

FIGURE 3-10 *Transient Neonatal Pustular Melanosis (TNPM)*
The biopsy shows a large subcorneal neutrophilic pustule in the center of the specimen. The dermis beneath the pustule contains an infiltrate of lymphocytes, histiocytes, and small numbers of neutrophils.

Erythema Toxicum Neonatarum

Erythema toxicum neonatarum is a common benign dermatosis that affects term infants within 12 to 48 hours after birth. Clinically, it presents with macular erythematous plaques and pustules especially on the face and trunk. It usually resolves in a few weeks, sometimes associated with blood eosinophilia (112, 113).

HISTOLOGY (FIGURE 3-11):
- Subcorneal or intraepidermal vesicles composed mainly of eosinophils (centered around a hair follicle)
- Sometimes neutrophilic infiltrate can be seen.
- Perivascular eosinophilic infiltrate

DIFFERENTIAL DIAGNOSIS:
- Incontinentia Pigmenti: Genodermatosis, almost always female infants. Histologically it has more dyskeratotic cells.
- Eosinophilic Pustular Folliculitis: Similar to erythema toxicum neonatarum histologically, but it has a completely different clinical presentation.
- Transient neonatal pustular melanosis and impetigo are not follicular in origin and the subcorneal vesicles are mainly composed of neutrophils.

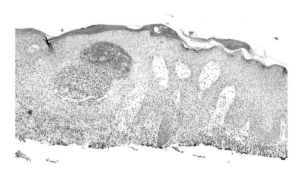

FIGURE 3-11 *Erythema Toxicum Neonatarum*
Intraepidermal vesicles with many neutrophils and eosinophils.

Bullous Pemphigoid

Bullous pemphigoid (BP) is an autoimmune bullous dermatosis disorder that usually affects elderly patients. BP is characterized by the presence of IgG autoantibodies specific for the hemidesmosomal BP antigens BP230 (BPAg1) and BP180 (BPAg2). Autoantibodies of BP target the NC16A domain of BPAg2 (lamina lucida) (also in pemphigoid gestationis and linear IgA lamina lucida type). Patients develop urticarial papules and plaques later associated with tense vesicles and bullae. The mucosal surfaces are less commonly affected. An uncommon variant, cicatricial pemphigoid, predominantly affects the skin of the head and neck and mucosal surfaces showing extensive scarring with skin involvement in only 25% of cases (114–118).

HISTOLOGY (FIGURE 3-12A, B):
- Urticarial lesions reveal a superficial perivascular mixed infiltrate composed of mononuclear cells and eosinophils. A helpful clue to the diagnosis of urticarial lesions is the presence of eosinophils in the basal cell layer of the epidermis, along with eosinophilic spongiosis.
- Biopsy of vesicles reveals a subepidermal blister associated with a variable mixed inflammatory infiltrate. Eosinophils, lymphocytes, and neutrophils in variable numbers within the bullae.
- DIF studies reveal linear deposition of IgG and C3 along the basement membrane. The salt-split skin test shows immunoreactants deposits in the roof of the blister, since this area contains the hemidesmosomes where the BPAg are located (lamina lucida) (**Figure 3-13A, B**).

DIFFERENTIAL DIAGNOSIS:
- The differential diagnosis includes other dermatoses with subepidermal bullae such as epidermolysis bullosa acquisita (EBA), herpes gestationis, and bullous drug eruption.
- EBA has very minimal inflammatory infiltrate and the salt-split skin test shows staining of the floor of the blister instead of the roof.
- Herpes gestationis shows similar findings to BP, but it occurs in pregnant women. DIF is identical to BP but IgG is present less often than C3 alone.
- Bullous drug eruption shows negative findings on DIF.
- Urticarial lesions of BP may resemble eczematous dermatitis, drug eruptions, etc.

Bullous Pemphigoid

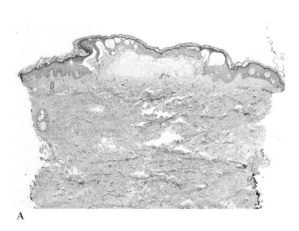
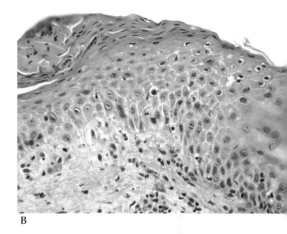

FIGURE 3-12 *Bullous Pemphigoid*
A. Subepidermal blister with eosinophils. **B.** Urticarial lesion of bullous pemphigoid showing eosinophilic spongiosis.

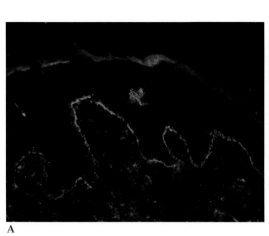
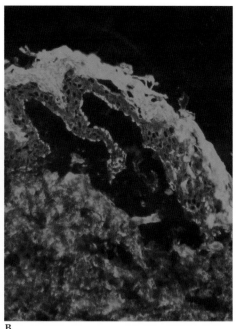

FIGURE 3-13 *Bullous Pemphigoid*
A. Direct immunofluorescence (DIF): Linear deposit of C3 along the basement membrane.
B. Direct immunofluorescence (DIF) with "salt split skin test": Linear deposit of C3 in the roof of the blister. (*Courtesy of Dr Matthew Fleming.*)

Cicatricial Pemphigoid

Cicatricial pemphigoid (CP) is characterized by scarring, with a predilection for mucosal surfaces. Most patients are elderly and males. Oral involvement is present in almost all patients. In the Brunsting-Perry variant there are no mucosal lesions but prominent erythematous patches with overlying recurrent blisters appear with atrophic scarring. DIF shows linear IgG and C3 in almost all cases identical to BP. The two major antigens associated with CP are BPAG2 (180 kD) and epiligrin (laminin-5). The autoantibodies from patients with CP target the C-terminal of BPAg2 (lamina lucida) (119–121).

HISTOLOGY (FIGURE 3-14):
- Subepidermal blister with neutrophils, lymphocytes, and histiocytes predominate in the inflammatory infiltrate (eosinophils sometimes are absent).
- Prominent fibrosis in dermis
- Oral lesions tend to have a prominent lichenoid infiltrate that is rich in eosinophils and neutrophils.

DIFFERENTIAL DIAGNOSIS:
- BP (see above)

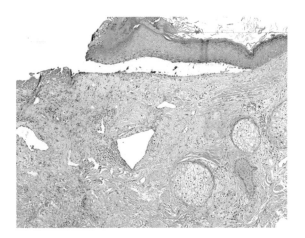

FIGURE 3-14 *Cicatricial Pemphigoid*
Subepidermal blister with scarring changes in dermis.

Pemphigoid Gestationis
(Herpes Gestationis)

Pemphigoid gestationis (PG) is a rare bullous eruption that occurs most commonly in the second or third trimester of pregnancy and in the postpartum period. The lesions start in the abdomen showing intense urticarial macules with subsequent involvement of the hands and feet. In the vast majority of patients with PG the autoimmune disease is directed to the NC16A domain of 180kD bullous pemphigoid antigen (BPAg2) (122–124).

HISTOLOGY (FIGURE 3-15):
- Subepidermal vesicle with variable mixed inflammatory infiltrate composed of lymphocytes, neutrophils, and eosinophils.
- The papillary dermis may be markedly edematous and necrotic keratinocytes can be seen in the basal layer.
- Early urticarial lesions show a mixed superficial perivascular infiltrate with eosinophilic spongiosis.
- DIF reveals a linear pattern with C3 along the DEJ in almost 100% of the cases, and IgG in 30% of cases.

DIFFERENTIAL DIAGNOSIS:
- BP (see above)
- Pruritic urticarial papules and plaques in pregnancy (PUPPP) is also associated with pregnancy, but rarely presents with blisters and DIF is negative.

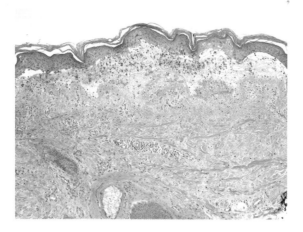

FIGURE 3-15 *Pemphigoid Gestationis* Subepidermal blister with lymphocytes, neutrophils, and eosinophils. Note the edema in superficial dermis.

Dermatitis Herpetiformis

Dermatitis herpetiformis (DH) is an immune-mediated blistering skin disease characterized by widespread, pruritic, papulovesicular erosions distributed symmetrically over the extensor surfaces of the extremities, scalp, shoulders, back, and buttocks. Inherited as an autosomal dominant trait, this disease usually presents in early adulthood but can be seen in all ages. DH shows histological evidence of celiac disease (gluten-sensitive enteropathy) in 90% of cases. There is evidence that the autoantigen in DH is a transglutaminase (TGase3) and that the skin lesions are caused by dermal deposition of circulating immune complexes containing both IgA and TGase3 (125–128).

HISTOLOGY (FIGURE 3-16A, B):
- Subepidermal papillary blisters with numerous neutrophils and variable numbers of eosinophils best seen in the erythematous phase away from the blister.
- The superficial dermis shows a mixed perivascular lymphocytic and neutrophilic infiltrate.
- The most characteristic feature is the presence of neutrophilic microabscesses associated with karyorrhexis within the tip of dermal papillae.
- DIF studies reveal granular deposits of IgA within the dermal papillae in the same distribution as the microabscesses. C3 can also be observed in the papillary dermis (**Figure 3-14C**).

DIFFERENTIAL DIAGNOSIS:
- Differential diagnosis includes linear IgA disease, BP, and bullous LE.
- Linear IgA usually affects children and can be very similar histologically, but usually has a linear arrangement of neutrophils at the dermal–epidermal junction and a linear pattern of IgA and C3 on DIF.
- Bullous LE shows subepidermal bullae with neutrophils and sometimes mucin deposition in dermis. DIF shows granular (40% of cases) or linear (60% of cases) deposition of multiple immunoreactants, including IgG, IgA, IgM, and C3.
- BP (see above)

Dermatitis Herpetiformis

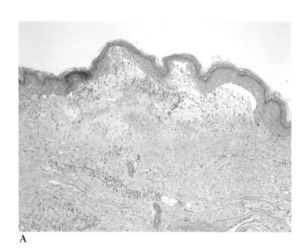

A

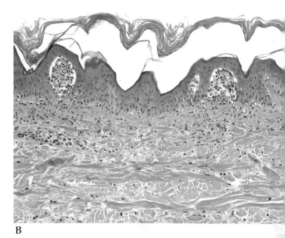

B

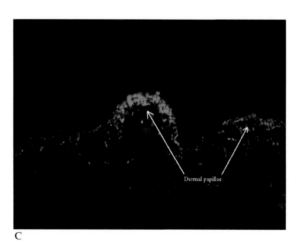

C

FIGURE 3-16 *Dermatitis Herpetiformis*
A. Subepidermal blister with many neutrophils. **B.** Neutrophilic microabscesses within the tip of dermal papillae. **C.** Direct immunofluorescence (DIF): Granular deposits of IgA within the dermal papillae in the same distribution as the microabscesses. (*Courtesy of Dr Matthew Fleming.*)

Linear IgA Dermatosis

Linear IgA dermatosis (LAD) includes linear IgA disease of adults and chronic bullous disease of childhood; they differ slightly in their clinical presentations but have identical immunopathologic features. LAD of adults is a rare disease that clinically presents with vesicles and bullae in a distribution similar to DH. Chronic bullous disease of childhood is characterized by vesicles and bullae with a predilection for perioral and genital regions. Like adult LAD, the childhood form may also be associated with blisters in an annular distribution ("cluster of jewels"). Both in adults and in children, LAD is frequently associated with mucous membrane involvement. Pathophysiology includes deposition of antigens within the dermal–epidermal junction, in different target sites, including the lamina lucida, the sublamina densa, or both simultaneously. Antibodies are more commonly found in the lamina lucida (rarely in sublamina densa), and are directed against the LAD-1 antigen in anchoring filaments (97 kD and 120 kD). Drug-induced LAD is usually associated with vancomycin, captopril, and somatostatin (129–132).

HISTOLOGY (FIGURE 3-17A):
■ Very similar to DH (sometimes identical)
■ Subepidermal blister with neutrophils
■ Less tendency to have papillary microabscesses formation and more tendency to form a uniform neutrophilic infiltration along the DEJ
■ DIF studies reveal linear deposition of IgA along the basement membrane in 100% of the patients, sometimes with deposition of complement (C3) (**Figure 3-15B**)

DIFFERENTIAL DIAGNOSIS:
■ DH (see above)
■ Can resemble BP sometimes (see above)

Linear IgA Dermatosis

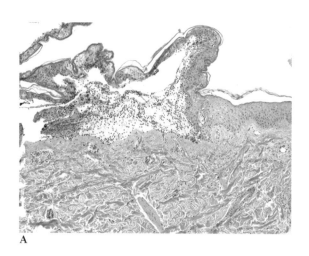

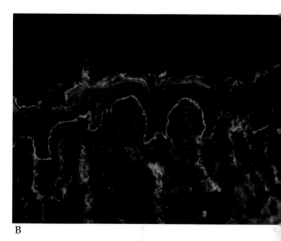

FIGURE 3-17 *Linear IgA Dermatosis*
A. Neutrophilic-rich subepidermal blister. **B.** Direct immunofluorescence (DIF): Linear deposits of IgA along the basement membrane. (*Courtesy of Dr Matthew Fleming.*)

Bullous Lupus Erythematosus

Bullous LE is a rare variant of lupus characterized by a widespread vesiculobullous eruption and with linear deposition of antibodies anti-basement membrane (collagen type VII). It usually arises in sun-exposed sites and is most often seen in young black women. Patients usually have a prior history of LE (133, 134).

HISTOLOGY (FIGURE 3-18):
- Subepidermal vesicles with numerous neutrophils and papillary dermal microabscesses similar to those seen in DH.
- Dermal mucin and the upper dermis show a perivascular mixed infiltrate composed of lymphocytes, eosinophils, and histiocytes.
- Vacuolar interface dermatitis.
- There may be leukocytoclastic vasculitis in the upper dermis.
- DIF shows granular (40% of cases) or linear (60% of cases) deposition of multiple immunoreactants, including IgG, IgA, IgM, and C3, and thus helps distinguish bullous LE from the other two subepidermal bullous disorders with a predominance of neutrophils (DH and LAD).

DIFFERENTIAL DIAGNOSIS:
- DH (see above)
- LAD (see above)

Bullous Lupus Erythematosus

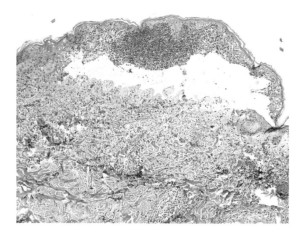

FIGURE 3-18 *Bullous Lupus Erythematosus*
Subepidermal vesicle with numerous
neutrophils.

Porphyria Cutanea Tarda

Porphyria cutanea tarda (PCT) is the most common type of porphyria, caused by a defect in uroporphyrinogen decarboxylase (URO-D) and inherited as an autosomal dominant trait. PCT includes familial types with URO-D gene mutations and acquired types (sporadic) with genetic predisposition after exposure to hepatotoxic agents (ethanol, estrogens, vitamin B12, etc.). Hepatitis C and AIDS infection have been associated with PCT. PCT is most commonly seen in young and middle-aged adults and is characterized by vesicles and bullae on sun-damaged skin, particularly the dorsum of the hands, face, and forearms. Vesicles frequently heal with scarring and milia formation. Hypertrichosis and hyperpigmentation of the face are common findings. Patients may have an increased risk of developing hepatocellular carcinoma (135–137).

HISTOLOGY (FIGURE 3-19A, B):
- Subepidermal blister with viable roof and festooning of the dermal papillae.
- Minimal to no inflammation (cell-poor lesions).
- Caterpillar bodies (linear eosinophilic basement membrane material) in the roof of the blister.
- Hyalinization of blood vessels in papillary dermis (PAS-positive).
- Solar elastosis is frequent.
- Late stage one can see dermal sclerosis.
- DIF shows IgG and C3 around dermal vessels and less staining at the DEJ in the lamina lucida.

DIFFERENTIAL DIAGNOSIS:
- Pseudoporphyria in patients with chronic renal failure or using some medications (furosemide, tetracycline, etc.). The histological and immunological findings are identical; however, these patients will show normal porphyrin metabolism.
- Similar histologic findings as in epidermolysis bullosa acquisita.

OTHER TYPES OF PORPHYRIA:
- **Acute Intermittent Porphyria (AIP):** Deficiency of porphobilinogen deaminase. Usually no skin lesions.
- **Congenital Erythropoietic Porphyria (CEP):** Deficiency of uroporphyrinogen III synthase deficiency. By histology it usually shows hyalinization in upper dermis.
- **Erythropoietic Protoporphyria (EPP):** Deficiency of ferrochelatase. Begins in childhood. By histology it usually shows prominent hyalinization in upper dermis and around superficial blood vessels (PAS +).
- **Variegate Porphyria:** Deficiency of protoporphyrinogen oxidase.
- **Hereditary Coproporphyria:** Coproporphyrinogen oxidase deficiency.

Porphyria Cutanea Tarda

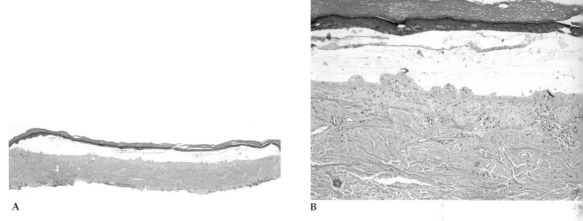

A   B

FIGURE 3-19 *Porphyria Cutanea Tarda*
A. Cell-poor subepidermal blister with festooning of the dermal papillae. **B.** Caterpillar bodies in the roof of the blister along with festooning of the dermal papillae.

Epidermolysis Bullosa

Epidermolysis bullosa (EB) represents a rare complex group of inherited mechano-bullous diseases with variable inheritance, clinical findings, and ultrastructural and molecular defects. There are three major groups of EB and numerous complex subclassification schemes; the three major categories are based on the level within the epidermis or basement membrane zone in which a blister is formed; these are the simplex, junctional, and dystrophic types of EB (138–142).

- **EB Simplex:** It is caused by an autosomal dominantly inherited defect in keratins 5 and 14 that result in cytolysis and vesicle formation. Although the vesicle appears to be subepidermal on routine histology, in fact the cleavage plane occurs within the cytoplasm of the basal cell layer. By EM, the roof of the bulla shows degenerative changes of the basal cells, a finding absent in other variants of EB. Immunohistochemistry allows detecting the fragments of basal keratinocytes still attached to the base of the blister (143). Several types of EB simplex have been recognized as Weber-Cockayne (localized), Koebner (generalized), EB simplex herpetiformis (Dowling-Meara), and muscular dystrophy type (only one with plectin defect).
- **Junctional EB:** It is inherited as an autosomal recessive trait associated with a defect in hemidesmosomes and anchoring filaments complex, laminin 5 or type XVII collagen (BPAg2, 180 kD), which results in a vesicle with a cleavage plane within the lamina lucida. The clinical expression of junctional EB ranges from a fairly benign disease to a severe condition that resembles dystrophic EB. Several types have been described; the pyloric atresia type is associated with alpha-6-beta-4 integrin defect.
- **EB Dystrophica:** It may be inherited as either an autosomal dominant or an autosomal recessive trait. This form of EB, which is typically more severe than the other groups, is caused by a defect in anchoring fibrils (type VII collagen) resulting in a subepidermal vesicle with a cleavage below the lamina densa. Associated with squamous cell carcinoma in 10% to 40% of patients.

HISTOLOGY:
- All forms of EB are characterized by a cell poor subepidermal vesicle.
- DIF is negative in all forms of EB except in EBA (see below).
- EM or immunohistochemistry (keratin, type IV collagen) may help determine the exact level of the blister (143).
- PAS stain may help determine if the basement membrane is located at the base or the roof of the blister (EB simplex or junctional/EB dystrophica, respectively).

DIFFERENTIAL DIAGNOSIS:
- Other cell poor subepidermal blistering diseases, such as PCT and EBA

Epidermolysis Bullosa Acquisita

Epidermolysis bullosa acquisita (EBA) is a rare non-inherited, chronic autoimmune subepidermal blistering disease of the skin and mucous membranes caused by antibodies directed against type VII collagen (below the sub-lamina densa). Patients with EBA are usually elderly and with slight female predominance. Clinically, it shows hemorrhagic vesicles on the backs of the hands that heal with scarring and milia similar to PCT (144–146).

HISTOLOGY (FIGURE 3-20):
- Cell-poor subepidermal blister
- Festooning of the dermal papillae in a pattern that mimics PCT
- Scarring and milia formation
- DIF labeling is usually required to distinguish EB from its mimics. DIF reveals linear distribution of IgG and C3 along the basement membrane region, just like in BP. In contrast, split skin immunofluorescence studies reveal deposition of immuno-reactants along the floor of the blister

DIFFERENTIAL DIAGNOSIS:
- BP, PCT (see above)

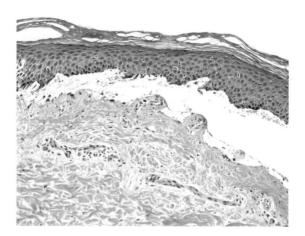

FIGURE 3-20 *Epidermolysis Bullosa Acquisita*
Cell-poor subepidermal blister similar to PCT.

Inflammatory Reactions Primarily Involving the Dermis and Subcutis

(*continued*)

(*continued*)

SARCOIDOSIS

FOREIGN BODY GRANULOMAS

CHEILITIS GRANULOMATOSA

MULTICENTRIC RETICULOHISTIOCYTOSIS

XANTHOGRANULOMA

BENIGN CEPHALIC HISTIOCYTOSIS

INTERSTITIAL GRANULOMATOUS DERMATITIS (PALISADED NEUTROPHILIC AND GRANULOMATOUS DERMATITIS)

VASCULITIS AND PURPURIC DISEASES

LEUKOCYTOCLASTIC VASCULITIS

GRANULOMA FACIALE

ERYTHEMA ELEVATUM DIUTINUM

POLYARTERITIS NODOSA

CHURG-STRAUSS SYNDROME (ALLERGIC GRANULOMATOSIS)

WEGENER GRANULOMATOSIS

PIGMENTED PURPURIC DERMATOSIS (CAPILLARITIS)

CRYOGLOBULINEMIA

DEGOS DISEASE (MALIGNANT ATROPHIC PAPULOSIS)

ATROPHIE BLANCHE (LIVEDOID VASCULITIS)

CALCIPHYLAXIS

SCURVY

SCLEROSING/FIBROSING DISORDERS INCLUDING OTHER DERMATOSIS OF CONNECTIVE TISSUE

MORPHEA/SCLERODERMA

NEPHROGENIC SYSTEMIC FIBROSIS

RADIATION DERMATITIS

PSEUDOXANTHOMA ELASTICUM

EOSINOPHILIC FASCIITIS (SHULMAN SYNDROME)

CONNECTIVE TISSUE NEVUS

FOCAL DERMAL HYPOPLASIA (GOLTZ SYNDROME)

KYRLE DISEASE (HYPERKERATOSIS FOLLICULARIS ET PARAFOLLICULARIS IN CUTEM PENETRANS)

ELASTOSIS PERFORANS SERPIGINOSA

PERFORATING FOLLICULITIS

REACTIVE PERFORATING COLLAGENOSIS

Drug Reactions

Drug reactions can present with almost any clinical and histological pattern. There are multiple histological and clinical variations.

Drug eruptions characterized by dermal hypersensitivity reaction:

■ The majority of patients with a reaction to a medication will develop a hypersensitivity reaction against the antigens that are delivered to the skin through the dermal vessels. Thus, they are usually characterized by infiltrates of lymphocytes and eosinophils around the superficial (and deep) dermal vascular plexus. The intervening dermis shows different degrees of edema. In general, there is little spongiosis, although some cases may develop significant spongiosis and increased numbers of dendritic cells (Langerhans cells) possibly indicating that some of the antigen reached the epidermis (147a).

HISTOLOGY:
■ Occasional spongiosis
■ Perivascular infiltrate of lymphocytes with scattered eosinophils
■ Dermal edema

Drug eruptions mainly characterized by interface dermatitis:

■ Exanthematous/Morbilliform Drug Reaction (See Interface Dermatitis section): most common type of drug reaction
■ Fixed drug eruption (see Interface Dermatitis section)
■ Lichenoid drug eruption (see Lichenoid/Vacuolar Interface Dermatitis section)
■ Erythema multiforme (see Interface Dermatitis section)

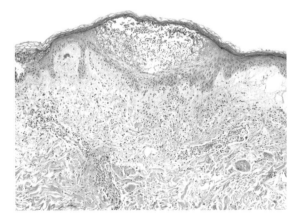

FIGURE 4-1 *Acute Generalized Exanthematous Pustulosis (AGEP)* Subcorneal pustule.

(continued)

Drug Reactions (*continued*)

The most common drug reactions show a predominantly lymphocytic infiltrate. However, there is a group with predominance of neutrophils:

- **Acute Generalized Exanthematous Pustulosis (AGEP):** Usually secondary to antibiotics administration. Histologically, it shows subcorneal and intraepidermal pustules; sometimes with LCV. The papillary dermis can be edematous and there is a dense mixed inflammatory response in the upper dermis with eosinophils (distinguishing feature from pustular psoriasis) (**Figure 4-1**). Differential diagnosis is with pustular psoriasis, subcorneal pustular dermatosis, Reiter disease, impetigo and dermatophytosis.
- **Drug-Induced Sweet Syndrome-Like Eruption:** Clinically and histologically identical to Sweet syndrome. Usually due to furosemide and oral contraceptive pills (OCP). A localized variation has been described as "neutrophilic dermatosis of the dorsal hands," which can show leukocytoclastic vasculitis.
- **Halogenoderma (Bromoderma):** Usually due to intake of bromides or iodides. Histologically, the lesions show pseudoepitheliomatous hyperplasia with intraepidermal microabscesses and granulomatous formation.

Drug eruptions characterized by bullae/vesicles:

- **Drug-Induced Pseudoporphyria:** Histologically identical to PCT. Usually due to antibiotics (ciprofloxacin), NSAIDs, and OCPs.
- **Drug-Induced Pemphigus:** Histologically identical to pemphigus vulgaris. Usually due to penicillamine. Penicillamine also can cause anetoderma (atrophy of the skin) and elastosis perforans serpiginosa.
- **Drug-Induced Linear IgA:** Histologically identical to linear IgA. Mainly due to vancomycin.

Drug-Induced hyperpigmentation:

- Associated drugs include minocycline (golden-brown pigment, positive for Perl stain and Fontana Masson in type II reactions), argyria, gold (black pigment), bleomycin, clofazimine (lipofuscin positive with PAS), and amiodarone (positive with PAS) (**Figure 4-2A–C**).

Other:

- **Drug-Induced Pseudolymphoma:** Histologically, lesions can be identical to mycosis fungoides. Associated drugs include phenytoin, carbamazepine, etc.
- **Neutrophilic Eccrine Hidradenitis:** Associated with chemotherapy. Histologically, one observes neutrophils surrounding and into eccrine ducts (**Figure 4-3**).
- **Chemotherapy-Induced Dermatitis:** Interface dermatitis with severe maturation arrest. The epidermis appears disorganized and keratinocytes are enlarged with pleomorphic nuclei and conspicuous nucleoli. Atypical mitosis within epidermis can be seen. Squamous metaplasia of the eccrine ducts (**Figure 4-4**).
- **Psoriasiform Drug Reactions:** Associated with beta-blockers Histologically identical to psoriasis.
- **Drug-Induced Vasculitis**

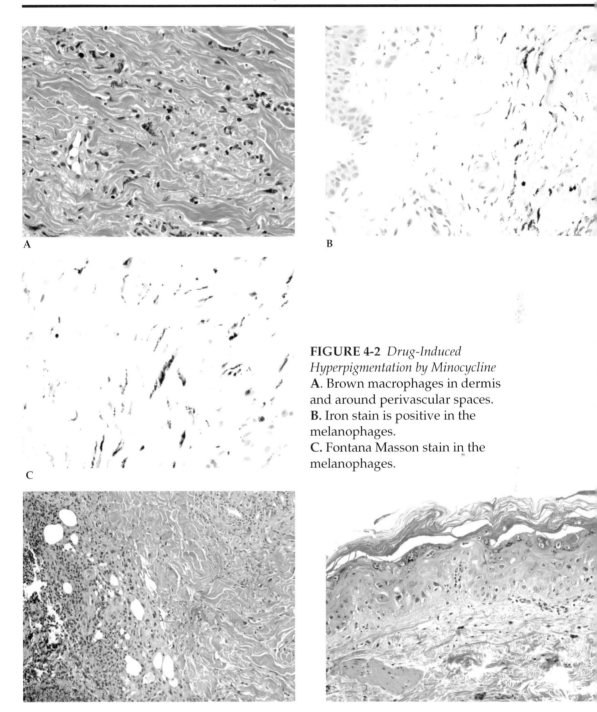

A

B

C

FIGURE 4-2 *Drug-Induced Hyperpigmentation by Minocycline*
A. Brown macrophages in dermis and around perivascular spaces.
B. Iron stain is positive in the melanophages.
C. Fontana Masson stain in the melanophages.

FIGURE 4-3 Neutrophilic eccrine hidradenitis. Dense neutrophilic inflammatory response around eccrine ducts.

FIGURE 4-4 Chemotherapy-induced dermatitis. Interface dermatitis with keratinocytes showing clear pleomorphism.

Urticaria

Urticaria is an IgE-mediated hypersensitivity reaction that is characterized clinically by the abrupt onset of raised erythematous lesions (wheals) that are often pruritic. Urticaria may be acute (lasting less than 6 weeks) or chronic (lasting more than 6 weeks) (147b, 148).

HISTOLOGY (FIGURE 4-5A, B):
- Normal epidermis
- Subtle perivascular and interstitial infiltrate composed of eosinophils, lymphocytes, neutrophils, and mast cells
- Dermal edema
- Dilated venules
- **Urticarial Vasculitis:** Leukocytoclastic vasculitis (**Figure 4-5C**)

DIFFERENTIAL DIAGNOSIS:
- Other types of hypersensitivity reactions, such as drug reaction

Urticaria

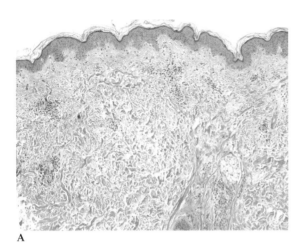

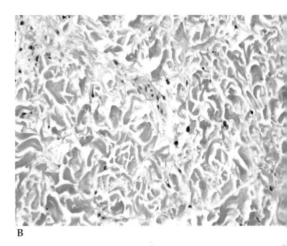

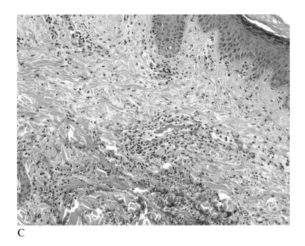

FIGURE 4-5 *Urticaria*
A. Subtle interstitial inflammatory response in dermis composed of lymphocytes, eosinophils, and neutrophils. Note the dermal edema. **B.** Higher magnification showing the interstitial cells in dermis (eosinophils and neutrophils). **C.** Urticarial vasculitis. Leukocytoclastic vasculitis with many eosinophils.

Urticaria Pigmentosa

It is the most common variant of mastocytosis. Clinically, it presents with multiple brown red macules mostly seen in children, and sometimes can show autosomal dominant mode of transmission with possible relationship to mutations in the KIT gene (Ckit) (149, 150).

HISTOLOGY (FIGURE 4-6A, B):
- Infiltrate in dermis (perivascular and interstitial) composed of mast cells
- Mast cells are characterized by the presence of metachromatic granules in their cytoplasm.
- Scattered eosinophils
- Special stains that may be used to highlight mast cells include Giemsa and Leder stain. To detect degranulated mast cells it may be better to use immunoperoxidase (e.g., with anti-ckit or anti-tryptase).

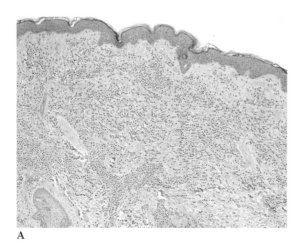
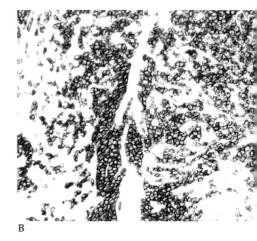

A   B

FIGURE 4-6 *Urticaria Pigmentosa*
A. Dense population of mast cells in dermis. **B.** Immunohistochemical studies with ckit (CD117) showing strong cytoplasmic and membranous positivity.

Telangectasia Macularis Eruptiva Perstans

Telangectasia macularis eruptiva perstans (TMEP) is usually seen in adults and is characterized by an extensive eruption of brown red macules with telangectasia. It has a high incidence of systemic involvement (151).

HISTOLOGY:
- Small number of mast cells limited to the upper third of the dermis and mainly located around dilated capillaries
- Diagnosis can be missed due to the small number of mast cells present in dermis. Special stains (Giemsa, Leder, or Toluidine blue) are helpful to make the correct diagnosis; however, they may fail to show degranulated mast cells. The latter are better identified with immunoperoxidase (e.g., with anti-ckit or anti-tryptase).

Postinflammatory Pigmentary Alteration

Postinflammatory pigmentary alteration (PPA) is a pigmentary alteration of the skin secondary to an inflammatory dermatosis, especially from dermatosis that affect the dermal-epidermal junction, such as lichen planus, benign lichenoid keratosis, fixed drug eruption, etc. Clinically it presents with either hypopigmented or hyperpigmented plaques (152).

HISTOLOGY (FIGURE 4-7):
- Presence of melanophages in superficial dermis
- Variable lymphocytic infiltrate of lymphocytes around blood vessels
- Sometimes with a focal residual interface damage and/or necrotic keratinocytes in papillary dermis

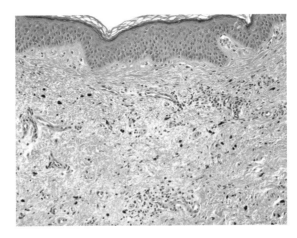

FIGURE 4-7 *Postinflammatory Pigmentary Alteration*
Increased number of melanophages in superficial dermis.

Erythema Dyschromicum Perstans

Erythema dyschromicum perstans (EDP) (also known as ashy dermatosis) presents clinically with bluish gray macules more commonly seen on the face and trunk. Most patients affected are Latino or Asian.

HISTOLOGY (FIGURE 4-8):
- Focal vacuolization of the basal layer
- The papillary dermis shows melanophages admixed with a subtle lymphohistiocytic infiltrate.
- Occasionally focal lymphocytic exocytosis

DIFFERENTIAL DIAGNOSIS:
- Late lesions of fixed drug eruption and PPA can show identical change; thus, clinical correlation is necessary.

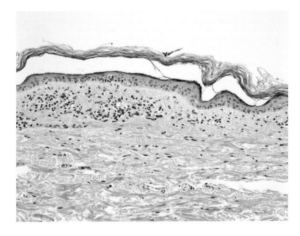

FIGURE 4-8 *Erythema Dyschromicum Perstans (Ashy Dermatosis)*
Subtle interface damage with scattered melanophages in superficial dermis.

Pruritic Urticarial Papules and Plaques of Pregnancy

Pruritic urticarial papules and plaques of pregnancy (PUPPP) is the most common rash seen in pregnancy, and it has predilection for primigravidas in the third trimester of pregnancy. Clinically, the rash starts in the abdomen and is characterized by pruritic erythematous urticarial papules, which can become vesicles. The rash usually involutes after pregnancy (153).

HISTOLOGY (FIGURE 4-9A, B):
- Mild spongiosis with parakeratosis
- Mild dermal edema
- Superficial and mid dermal perivascular lymphohistiocytic infiltrate admixed with rare eosinophils and neutrophils

DIFFERENTIAL DIAGNOSIS:
- PUPPP is mainly biopsied to rule out pemphigoid gestationis, which usually shows a subepidermal vesicle with variable mixed inflammatory infiltrate composed of lymphocytes, neutrophils, and eosinophils. Also, DIF is negative in PUPPP.

Pruritic Urticarial Papules and Plaques of Pregnancy

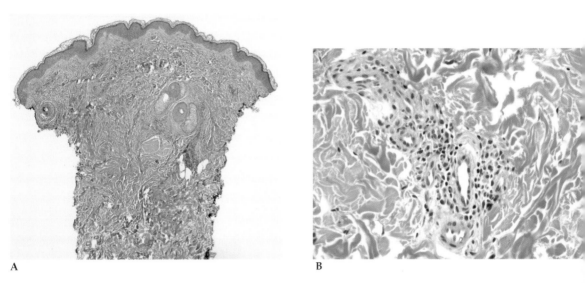

A   B

FIGURE 4-9 *Pruritic Urticarial Papules and Plaques of Pregnancy (PUPPP)*
A. Mild epidermal spongiosis with a superficial perivascular lymphocytic infiltrate admixed with rare eosinophils. **B.** High power showing a perivascular lymphocytic infiltrate with eosinophils.

Arthropod Assault ("Insect Bite") Reaction

We prefer the term originally coined by Dr. Christopher Shea of "arthropod assault" rather than "insect bite" since not all offending organisms are insects and not all are bites. The underlying mechanism is usually that of a delayed hypersensitivity reaction, resulting in a spectrum of clinical lesions ranging from urticaria to firm red nodules. Some insect bites, especially those caused by fleas, mosquitoes, and bedbugs, result in clinical lesions sometimes called papular urticaria. Reactions to arthropods will vary in their histologic appearance depending upon the capacity of host response, age of the lesion, and the type of the offending arthropod (154, 155).

HISTOLOGY (FIGURE 4-10A, B):
■ Epidermal hyperplasia (sometimes with intraepidermal necrosis or vesicles)
■ Spongiosis
■ Superficial and deep perivascular lymphohistiocytic infiltrate with eosinophils and plasma cells (predominance of neutrophils in spider bites)
■ Rarely, some lesions may show a subepidermal blister with eosinophils (bullous arthropod bite reaction).
■ Some lesions may have scattered large, CD30-positive lymphocytes.

DIFFERENTIAL DIAGNOSIS:
■ Other types of hypersensitivity reactions
■ Bullous Arthropod Bite Reaction: Bullous pemphigoid, bullous drug, linear IgA (rarely), dermatitis herpetiformis (rarely)
■ Lymphomatoid papulosis

Arthropod Assault ("Insect Bite") Reaction

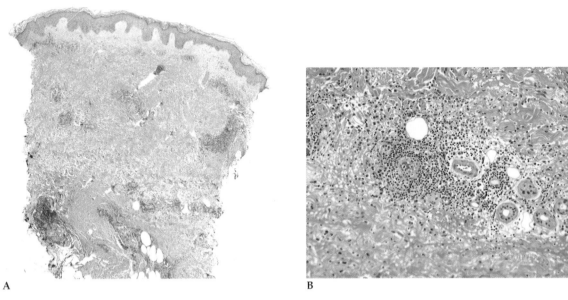

A

B

FIGURE 4-10 *Arthropod Assault ("Insect Bite") Reaction*
A. Dense superficial and deep perivascular dermatitis with eosinophilia. **B.** Higher magnification a dense perivascular lymphocytic infiltrate admixed with many eosinophils, which also extend into the adjacent interstitial dermis.

Polymorphous Light Eruption

Polymorphous light eruption (PMLE) is a common photoinduced eruption that clinically is characterized by recurrent delayed reactions to sunlight, ranging from erythematous papules, papulovesicles, and plaques to erythema multiforme-like lesions on sun-exposed surfaces. These lesions often develop within 30 minutes to 3 days after ultraviolet exposure and resolve in up to 10 days (156).

HISTOLOGY (FIGURE 4-11):
- Mild spongiosis
- Rare dyskeratotic keratinocytes
- Subepidermal edema
- Superficial and deep perivascular lymphocytic infiltrate (only a superficial perivascular pattern in early lesions)

DIFFERENTIAL DIAGNOSIS:
- Histologically, PMLE must be differentiated from lupus erythematosus (LE) and Jessner lymphocytic infiltrate (some authors consider Jessner a type of tumid lupus).
- In LE, there is prominent interface vacuolar damage in epidermis and papillary edema is not a feature. In addition, dermal mucin deposition is not a feature of PMLE.
- In Jessner lymphocytic infiltrate there are no changes within epidermis and no subepidermal edema.

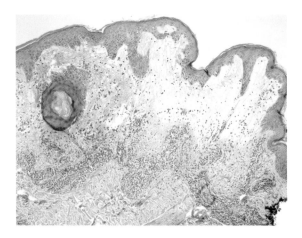

FIGURE 4-11 *Polymorphous Light Eruption (PMLE)* Subepidermal edema with a dense superficial perivascular lymphocytic infiltrate.

Gyrate Erythemas

These are a heterogeneous group of dermatoses that include erythema annulare centrifugum (EAC), erythema chronicum migrans (ECM) (Lyme disease), erythema gyratum repens (EGR) (associated with underlying internal malignancies), etc. (157, 158).

HISTOLOGY (FIGURE 4-12A, B):

- **EAC:** Focal spongiosis with parakeratosis and a demarcated coat sleeve-like lymphocytic infiltrate localized around the dilated superficial and deep blood vessels. The superficial variant of EAC shows only a superficial perivascular lymphocytic infiltrate and can show basilar vacuolar damage of keratinocytes. Also, the superficial variant may show extravasated red blood cells in superficial dermis (pityriasiform spongiosis) thus very similar to pityriasis rosea.
- **ECM:** Focal spongiosis with perivascular lymphocytic infiltrate often admixed with plasma cells and eosinophils. Sometimes there is endothelial swelling accompanied by variable dermal mucin deposition and perineural lymphocytic infiltrate.
- **EGR:** Spongiosis with parakeratosis, focal mild perivascular lymphocytic infiltrate, variable edema and with occasional eosinophilia of the dermis.

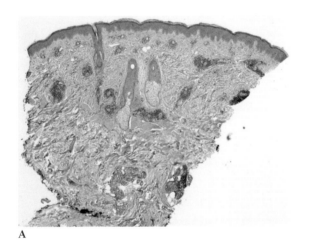 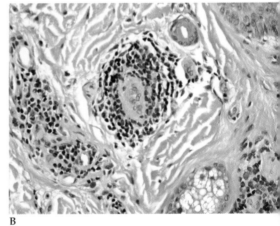

A   B

FIGURE 4-12 *Erythema Annulare Centrifugum*
A. Marked coat sleeve-like lymphocytic infiltrate around superficial and deep blood vessels. Epidermis shows mild spongiosis. **B.** Higher magnification shows a coat-sleeve lymphocytic infiltrate around blood vessels.

Perniosis (Chilblains)

Perniosis is an inflammatory dermatosis that presents after exposure to cold. Clinically, manifests as pruritic and/or painful erythematous-to-violaceous nodular or papular acral lesions (also can be seen in the buttock and thigh).

HISTOLOGY (FIGURE 4-13):
- Dense superficial and deep perivascular lymphocytic infiltrate (exocytosis to the acrosyringium)
- Occasional epidermal edema and/or necrosis
- Papillary edema
- Edema of blood vessels wall with transmural lymphocytic infiltrate ("fluffy edema" characteristic)
- Thrombi may be noted in superficial dermis
- Mucin around eccrine coil

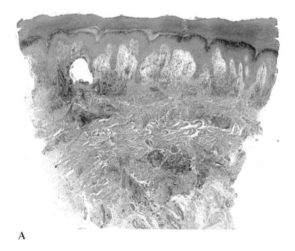 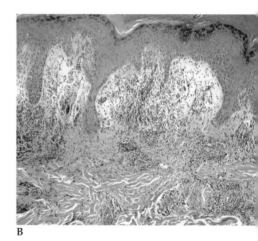

A   B

FIGURE 4-13 *Perniosis*
A. Dense superficial and deep perivascular lymphocytic infiltrate with marked papillary edema. **B.** Higher magnification showing a marked subepidermal edema with lymphocytic exocytosis.

Acute Febrile Neutrophilic Dermatosis
(Sweet Syndrome)

This is a reactive process that occurs in response to systemic factors, such as hematologic disease, infection, inflammation, vaccination, or drug exposure. Clinically, it is characterized by the abrupt onset of tender, red-to-purple papules, and nodules that are usually located on upper extremities, face, or neck and are typically accompanied by fever and peripheral neutrophilia (159–161).

HISTOLOGY (FIGURE 4-14A, B):
■ Diffuse dermal neutrophilic infiltrate in dermis admixed with histiocytes, plasma cells, and eosinophils (sometimes extravasated red blood cells)
■ Leukocytoclastic nuclear debris is classically present
■ Focal spongiosis (sometimes necrosis and subepidermal blister)
■ Superficial dermal edema
■ Very rarely vasculitis

DIFFERENTIAL DIAGNOSIS:
■ The differential diagnosis of Sweet syndrome includes other dermatosis with neutrophilic inflammation in dermis such as infectious diseases, rheumatoid neutrophilic dermatosis, pyoderma gangrenosum, Behcet disease, bowel bypass syndrome, vasculitis, etc. Clinical correlation is of paramount importance to distinguish these disorders.

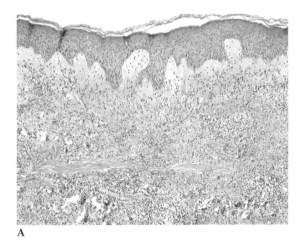 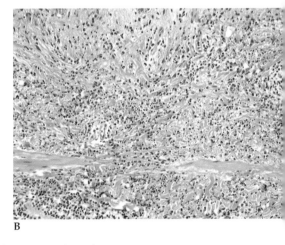

A   B

FIGURE 4-14 *Acute Febrile Neutrophilic Dermatosis (Sweet Syndrome)*
A. Diffuse neutrophilic inflammation in dermis with subepidermal papillary edema.
B. Higher magnification showing dense neutrophilic inflammation in dermis with leukocytoclastic nuclear debris and without vasculitis.

Pyoderma Gangrenosum

Pyoderma gangrenosum (PG) is an uncommon ulcerative cutaneous condition of uncertain etiology that has been associated with several diseases such as inflammatory bowel disease (ulcerative colitis or Crohn disease), arthritis, leukemia, predominantly myelocytic in nature or monoclonal gammopathies (IgA), etc. Clinically, it presents with ulcers with ragged, undermined violaceous edge classically located on the lower extremities (162, 163).

HISTOLOGY:
- Necrotic/ulcerated epidermis
- Diffuse neutrophilic infiltrate in dermis (sometimes extending into subcutis)
- Leukocytoclastic vasculitis occasionally
- In early disease, there may be a mixed cell infiltrate

DIFFERENTIAL DIAGNOSIS:
- PG is a primarily clinical diagnosis after excluding other causes of ulcers such as infectious diseases, etc. Always perform special stains to rule out infectious organisms.
- Sweet syndrome is not associated with ulceration and shows prominent karyorrhexis.

Well Syndrome
(Eosinophilic Cellulitis)

It is an uncommon condition that clinically presents with a mildly pruritic or tender cellulitis-like eruption with often blister formation. Well syndrome is usually sporadic, but there have been some familial cases. It is usually idiopathic but some cases are associated with hypersensitivity reactions to an arthropod bite or sting, cutaneous viral infections, leukemia, medications, etc. (164).

HISTOLOGY (FIGURE 4-15A, B):
- Spongiosis with intraepidermal or subepidermal blisters
- Diffuse dermal eosinophils in dermis admixed with histiocytes and lymphocytes
- Flame figures (collections of eosinophils with eosinophilic granules) and edema in dermis

DIFFERENTIAL DIAGNOSIS:
- Eosinophilic dermal infiltrates with flame figure formation can be seen in a number of conditions including arthropod reactions, drug reactions, bullous pemphigoid, fungal infections, allergic eczemas, eosinophilic folliculitis (clusters of degranulated eosinophils resulting in hypereosinophilic collagen), hypereosinophilic syndrome, etc.

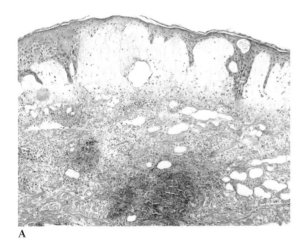
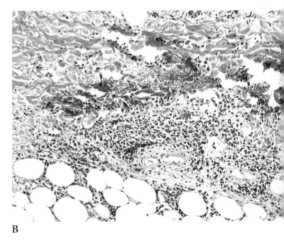

A   B

FIGURE 4-15 *Well Syndrome (Eosinophilic Cellulitis)*
A. Diffuse dermal infiltrate of eosinophils, histiocytes, and eosinophilic debris between collagen bundles forming flame figures. **B.** Higher magnification of collections of eosinophils with eosinophilic granules forming "flame figures."

Granuloma Annulare

Granuloma annulare (GA) is a common, self-limited, benign dermatosis characterized clinically by dermal papules and annular plaques. Localized GA is the common-
est variant and is characterized by multiple red annular lesions usually located in
acral sites. The generalized form of GA presents with pink to violaceous translucent
lichenoid papules diffusely involving the trunk and flexor surfaces of the extremities.
Subcutaneous GA is characterized by firm, flesh-colored nodules usually seen on the
extremities (frequently near joints) in young children. Perforating GA is characterized
by umbilicated papules most commonly located on the extremities of children. Apart
from the most common idiopathic form, GA is sometimes associated with HIV, herpes
zoster, tattoos, lymphoma, and sarcoidosis (165–167).

HISTOLOGY (FIGURE 4-16A, B):
- Palisading granulomas with necrobiotic collagen
- Mucin deposition
- Chronic inflammatory response surrounding the areas of necrobiosis
- Giant cells (rarely)
- Superficial and deep perivascular inflammatory cell infiltrate (lymphocytes, histio-
  cytes, and eosinophils) away from the necrobiotic areas
- Interstitial GA reveals only scattered macrophages lining brightly eosinophilic
  collagen within a mucinous background (**Figure 4-16C, D**)

DIFFERENTIAL DIAGNOSIS:
- Rheumatoid nodule and necrobiosis lipoidica can simulate GA.
- In contrast with necrobiosis lipoidica, GA has abundant mucin and lacks the characteristic layered pattern and multinucleated giant cells.
- In contrast with rheumatoid nodule, GA has prominent mucin and lacks the prominent fibrin deposition.
- In young adults on the distal extremities the differential diagnosis includes epithelioid sarcoma. The latter has more prominent cytologic atypia and the tumor cells
  express keratin.

Granuloma Annulare

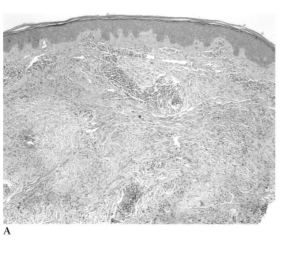

A

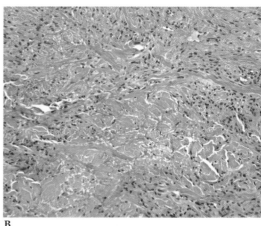

B

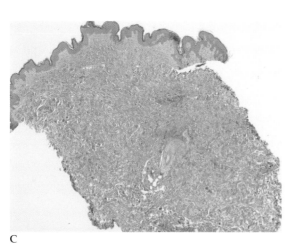

C

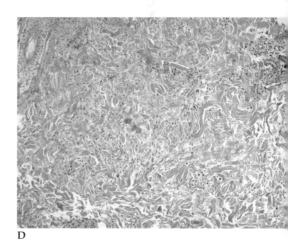

D

FIGURE 4-16 *Granuloma Annulare*
A. Necrobiotic collagen with peripheral palisading histiocytes. Note the focal mucin deposition along with the subtle surrounding chronic inflammatory response.
B. Higher magnification showing the necrobiotic collagen and the increased number of peripheral and interstitial histiocytes. Note the rare eosinophils. **C.** Interstitial granuloma annulare. The changes are very subtle. Note the busy dermis with increased number of histiocytes and inflammatory cells. **D.** Interstitial granuloma annulare. Higher magnification shows the histiocytes arranged about vessels and between collagen bundles that are separated by dermal mucin.

Annular Elastolytic Granuloma (Actinic Granuloma of O'Brien)

Annular elastolytic granuloma is a localized chronic dermatosis consisting of slowly enlarging annular plaques on sun-exposed areas. Some authors consider this lesion to be a form of granuloma annulare involving sun-exposed skin. The most common sites are the face, scalp, neck, and arms (168).

HISTOLOGY (FIGURE 4-17A, B):

- ◾ Granulomatous reaction within mid dermis composed of epithelioid macrophages, lymphocytes, and giant cells among the altered collagen bundles
- ◾ Multinucleated giant cells with intracytoplasmic blue-gray elastotic fibers (elastophagocytosis)
- ◾ Asteroid bodies (rarely)

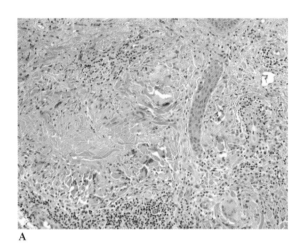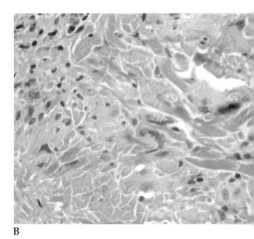

A   B

FIGURE 4-17 *Annular Elastolytic Granuloma*
A. Granuloma annulare-like reaction with increased number of giant cells engulfing elastotic material. **B.** Higher magnification showing the elastophagocytosis.

Necrobiosis Lipoidica

Necrobiosis lipoidica (NL) is a chronic granulomatous dermatosis characterized by one or more yellow-brown, telangiectatic plaques with central atrophy and raised violaceous borders typically on the pretibial regions. NL has been associated with diabetes mellitus (DM) in up to 11% of the cases, hence the term "necrobiosis lipoidica diabeticorum" sometimes used for this disease; other associations are sarcoidosis, hypo- or hyperthyroidism, systemic vasculitis, and inflammatory bowel disease, etc. (169, 170).

HISTOLOGY (FIGURE 4-18A, B):

- Presence of palisading necrobiotic granulomas in the lower two thirds of the reticular dermis, arranged parallel to the epidermis in a "layer cake" pattern
- Areas of degenerated collagen appear eosinophilic and hyalinized.
- Lipid-filled multinucleated giant cells
- Superficial and deep perivascular lymphocytic infiltrate with many plasma cells
- Subcutaneous involvement results in a pattern of septal panniculitis.

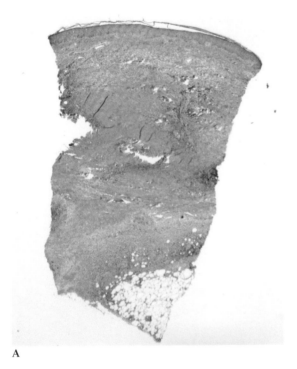

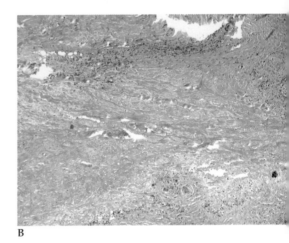

A   B

FIGURE 4-18 *Necrobiosis Lipoidica*
A. Degeneration of collagen bundles in a laminated pattern (layer cake) extending in the subcutaneous fat. **B.** Higher magnification showing the areas of degenerated collagen arranged in a layer cake pattern.

Necrobiotic Xanthogranuloma

Necrobiotic xanthogranuloma (NXG) is a rare condition of unknown etiology characterized by the presence of papules and nodules that show a predilection to the periorbital area. Most patients with NXG have an associated monoclonal paraproteinemia (usually IgG kappa type). Other associations include diabetes mellitus, multiple myeloma, B-cell lymphoma, etc. (171).

HISTOLOGY (FIGURE 4-19A, B):
- Xanthogranulomatous infiltration in mid dermis along with extensive areas of necrobiosis extending into the subcutaneous tissue
- The granulomatous infiltrate shows epithelioid and foamy histiocytes.
- Numerous giant cells (Touton and foreign-body giant cells not uncommon)
- Giant cells with bizarre and angulated morphology
- Chronic inflammatory response are a prominent feature (lymphocytes and plasma cells).
- Cholesterol clefts are often seen within the foci of necrobiosis and xanthogranulomatous inflammation.

DIFFERENTIAL DIAGNOSIS:
- The main differential diagnosis is with necrobiosis lipoidica, which should be distinguished clinically and histologically. The anatomic site (periorbital) plus the histomorphologic changes including the absence of massive necrobiosis, presence of cholesterol clefts, bizarre multinucleated giant cells, and Touton giant cells are in favor of NXG.

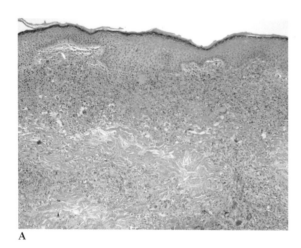 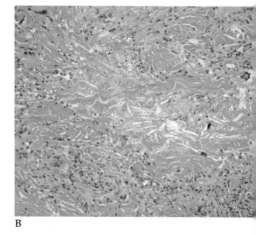

A   B

FIGURE 4-19 *Necrobiotic Xanthogranuloma (NXG)*
A. The biopsy shows a xanthogranulomatous infiltration in dermis with necrotic areas. **B.** Areas of necrobiosis with many foamy macrophages and cholesterol clefts.

Rheumatoid Nodule

Rheumatoid nodules are subcutaneous lesions often seen in approximately 30% of patients with rheumatoid arthritis. Similar nodules may occur in patients with rheumatic fever, rare cases of SLE (5–7%), and in seronegative ankylosing spondylitis. Lesions usually occur over the extensor aspect of forearms and elbows, back, scalp, feet, etc. (169, 172).

HISTOLOGY (FIGURE 4-20):
- The lesions are multinodular showing a central necrotic zone of amorphous, eosinophilic, fibrinoid material surrounded by a crown of palisading histiocytes and lymphocytes.
- The lesions primarily involve the subcutaneous fat and may extend into the deep dermis.
- Lack mucin deposition

DIFFERENTIAL DIAGNOSIS:
- The main differential of rheumatoid nodule is with subcutaneous (deep) granuloma annulare (pseudorheumatoid nodule). In rheumatoid nodule there is absence of mucin and instead there are prominent fibrinoid changes. Special stains (mucin) sometimes can be of help.

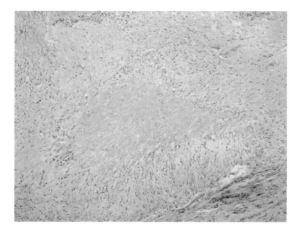

FIGURE 4-20 *Rheumatoid Nodule*
Palisading granulomatous changes with a central area of fibrinoid changes that lacks mucin deposition.

Rheumatic Fever Nodule

Rheumatic fever nodules are subcutaneous nodules found in approximately one third of patients with rheumatic fever. Lesions are small (2 to 3 mm), multiple, with a tendency to occur over bone prominences such as knuckles, olecranon processes, and humeral epicondyles (169).

HISTOLOGY:
- The lesions involve the deep dermis or subcutaneous tissue.
- Lace-like fibrin deposition and focal alteration of collagen admixed with neutrophils, lymphocytes, and karyorrhexis
- The nodules can be surrounded by prominent blood vessels.

Sarcoidosis

Sarcoidosis is a multisystemic disease in which cutaneous lesions can be seen in 10%-35% of cases. Also, cutaneous lesions may be the only manifestation of the disease. Lesions may be non-specific or specific. The non-specific lesions include erythema nodosum, erythema multiforme, etc. The specific lesions include non-caseating granuloma in dermis (173, 174).

HISTOLOGY (FIGURE 4-21):
- Dense non-caseating granulomas in dermis (sometimes they can extend to the subcutaneous tissue)
- Granulomas are uniform in size and shape.
- Granulomas are composed of epithelioid histiocytes admixed with variable number of Langhans giant cells.
- Small areas of fibrinoid necrosis
- Schaumann and asteroid bodies (not pathognomonic)
- No or only mild surrounding lymphocytic infiltrate
- Foreign polarizable material in up to 5% of cases

DIFFERENTIAL DIAGNOSIS:
- Sarcoidosis is a diagnosis of exclusion. Dermatoses that should be excluded include infections (tuberculosis, leprosy, fungal infections, etc.), Crohn disease, berylliosis, foreign body granulomas, etc. Labial and gingival involvement can be mistaken for Crohn disease and granulomatous cheilitis.

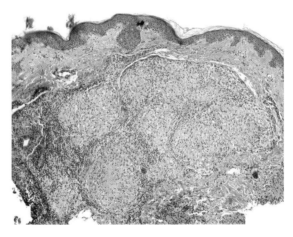

FIGURE 4-21 *Sarcoidosis*
Non-caseating granulomas in dermis surrounded by sparse lymphocytic inflammation.

Foreign Body Granulomas

Foreign body granulomas are a reaction to exogenous or endogenous materials that are too large to be ingested by macrophages. These substances can sometimes induce a granulomatous reaction that then mimics primary granulomatous disorders. In most cases, foreign material can be recognized in H&E sections; however, in some cases polarized light should be used to identify the birefringent foreign material.

HISTOLOGY:
- Caseating or non caseating granulomas
- Beryllium (fluorescent light bulbs) and zirconium (deodorants) can mimic sarcoidosis (naked granulomas). Spectrographic analysis may be used to confirm the diagnosis.
- Starch: "Maltese cross"; PAS and GMS positive
- Talc and Silica: Doubly refractile
- Suture Material: Birefringent refractile, multicolored
- Tattoo Material: Most tattoos appear black with granulomatous reaction.
- Exogenous lipids can form a "Swiss cheese" appearance in dermis. Paraffinomas occur after injection of oils, vitamin E, or grease. Sclerosing lipogranulomas can occur in the male genitalia after injection of paraffin or oil.
- Wood Splinter: Appears brown in color, sometimes with fungi (especially dematiacious fungi)
- Monsel Tattoo: Brown-black deposits in dermis from the use of ferrous sulfate for hemostasis (sometimes it can resemble a melanocytic lesion) (**Figure 4-22**)

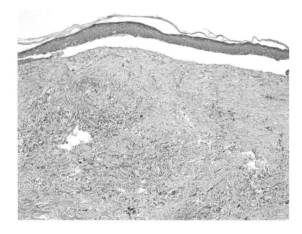

FIGURE 4-22 *Monsel Tattoo*
Note in increased number of pigmented macrophages.

Cheilitis Granulomatosa

This is a chronic swelling of the lip due to non-caseating granulomatous inflammation. Melkerson-Rosenthal syndrome is a rare triad of facial nerve palsy, fissured tongue (lingua plicata) and cheilitis granulomatosa (175). Many etiologies have been associated with cheilitis granulomatosa including infections (Mycobacterium, Borrelia, etc.), hypersensitivity reactions (food, fragances, etc.).

HISTOLOGY (FIGURE 4-23):
- Non-caseating granulomas in lamina propria adjacent to lymphatic vessels (sometimes the granulomas are small and poorly formed)
- Interstitial and nodular infiltrate of lymphocytes and plasma cells
- Edematous stroma

DIFFERENTIAL DIAGNOSIS:
- Non-caseating granulomas in this clinical setting are histologically indistinguishable from metastatic Crohn disease.
- Sarcoidosis tend to form larger granulomas and lack a dense lymphocytic infiltrate.

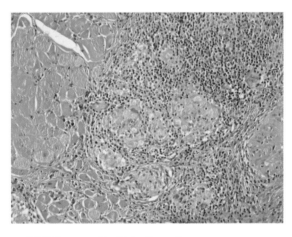

FIGURE 4-23 *Cheilitis Granulomatosa*
Non-caseating granulomas admixed with a dense lymphoplasmacytic inflammation.

Multicentric Reticulohistiocytosis

Multicentric reticulohistiocytosis (MRH) is a rare systemic disease of unknown etiology characterized by mucocutaneous papulonodules and erosive mutilating arthritis. MRH is paraneoplastic in about 30% of the cases (176, 177).

HISTOLOGY (FIGURE 4-24A, B):
- Nodular infiltrate of histiocytes with ample eosinophilic cytoplasm (ground glass).
- Bizarre multinucleated giant cells
- A mixed inflammatory response (lymphocytes, plasma cells, eosinophils)
- PAS-positive cytoplasm
- **Reticulohistiocytoma:** Same histology but a solitary nodule without systemic disease

DIFFERENTIAL DIAGNOSIS:
- The main differential diagnosis is with juvenile xanthogranuloma (JXG), which is seen in younger patients and histologically differs by the presence of Touton giant cells and lack of ground-glass cytoplasm.

Multicentric Reticulohistiocytosis

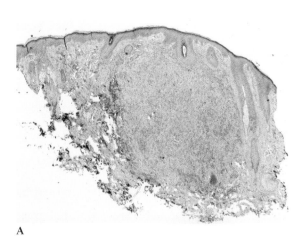

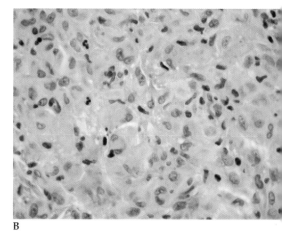

A

B

FIGURE 4-24 *Multicentric Reticulohistiocytosis*
A. Nodular population of macrophages with eosinophilic, finely granular (ground glass) cytoplasm. **B.** Higher magnification shows the histiocytic cells with eosinophils cytoplasm (ground glass appearance).

Xanthogranuloma

Xanthogranuloma (XG) is a benign, usually asymptomatic, solitary, self-healing nodule that predominantly occurs in infancy and childhood (first 5 years of life), thus some authors designate it as Juvenile Xanthogranuloma but sometimes can be seen in adults. The most common location is the head and neck area, followed by the upper extremities and trunk. Multiple XG and café-au-lait macules can be indicative of neurofibromatosis Type 1. Other associations include juvenile myelomonocytic leukemia and the prevalence is especially high in patients with coexistent neurofibromatosis (178, 179).

HISTOLOGY (FIGURE 4-25A, B):
■ Ill-defined dense intradermal monomorphous histiocytes forming a nodule and sometimes a diffuse infiltrate
■ Common mixed inflammatory infiltrate composed of lymphocytes, neutrophils, eosinophils, and mast cells (rarely)
■ Characteristic Touton and foreign body giants cells
■ Nuclear atypia and mitoses in up to 10% of cases
■ Older lesions tend to have increased amount of fibrosis
■ By IHC the histiocytes are positive for CD45, CD4, CD68, HAM-56, Factor XIIIA (negative for CD1a)
■ Sometimes the cells can be focally positive for S100p.

DIFFERENTIAL DIAGNOSIS:
■ Xanthomas usually lack inflammatory response and Touton giant cells.
■ Langerhans cell histiocytosis usually infiltrates the epidermis, lacks Touton giant cells, and has a more intense eosinophilic infiltrate.
■ Reticulohistiocytoma can be difficult to differentiate it from XG and the presence of large ground glass histiocytes with PAS-positive cytoplasm favors the diagnosis of reticulohistiocytoma.
■ XG may be confused with dermatofibroma especially in older lesions with increased amount of fibrosis. In such instances, IHC studies can be of help since cells in DF are negative for both CD45 and CD4.

Xanthogranuloma

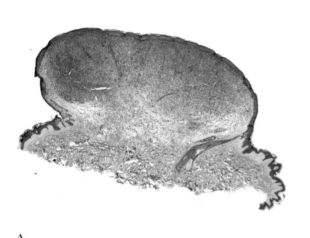

A

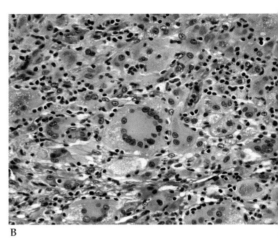

B

FIGURE 4-25 *Xanthogranuloma (XG)*
A. Polypoid growth of macrophages admixed with Touton giant cells. **B.** Higher magnification showing a mixture of Touton giant cells, macrophages, and lymphocytes.

Benign Cephalic Histiocytosis

Benign cephalic histiocytosis (BCH) is a rare histiocytosis of unknown etiology that presents early in childhood (between 3 months and 34 months). Clinically, the lesions are round/oval maculopapules more commonly seen around the face. BCH is associated with spontaneous regression (180).

HISTOLOGY:
- Histiocytic infiltrate in upper dermis
- The histiocytes are large with abundant eosinophilic cytoplasm.
- Mixture of eosinophils and lymphocytes are commonly seen.
- The histiocytes can rarely display pleomorphism.
- By IHC studies the histiocytes express CD68 and HAM-56 and negative for S100p and CD1a.

DIFFERENTIAL DIAGNOSIS:
- The main differential diagnosis is with Langerhans cell histiocytosis and can be differentiated by the presence in the latter of epidermal involvement and the expression both S100p and CD1a.

Interstitial Granulomatous Dermatitis (Palisaded Neutrophilic and Granulomatous Dermatitis)

Interstitial granulomatous dermatitis (IGD) is a histologic inflammatory reaction pattern with a large differential diagnosis that requires clinicopathologic correlation to identify the underlying cause. Clinically, it presents as linear or arciform subcutaneous cords, papules, or plaques. IGD is typically associated with autoimmune or connective-tissue disorders, such as rheumatoid arthritis, systemic lupus erythematosus, Wegener granulomatosis, systemic vasculitis, and also with lymphoproliferative disorders (181, 182).

HISTOLOGY (FIGURE 4-26A, B):
- Early lesions show increased number of neutrophils in dermis along with collagen degeneration.
- Occasional leukocytoclastic vasculitis and dermal mucin
- Developed lesions show granuloma annulare-like pattern, with an interstitial and perivascular infiltrate or neutrophils, lymphocytes and histiocytes (rare eosinophils) and necrobiotic collagen.
- Late lesions show granulomas with palisading histiocytes around basophilic collagen fibers (fibrin deposition) and scattered neutrophils.

DIFFERENTIAL DIAGNOSIS:
- Granuloma annulare is the main differential diagnosis but usually does not show neutrophils/leukocytoclasia.
- The histologic changes of IGD may be identical to rheumatoid nodules and rheumatic fever nodules.
- Interface dermatitis in association with palisading granulomatous changes may be observed in drug reactions, as with beta-blockers, angiotensin-converting enzyme inhibitors, and calcium channel blockers.

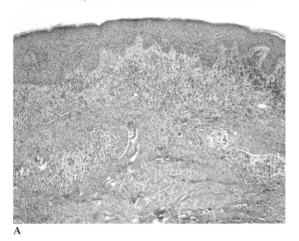 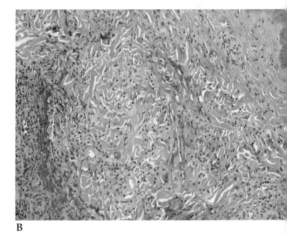

A   B

FIGURE 4-26 *Interstitial Granulomatous Dermatitis*
A. The biopsy shows an increased number of neutrophils in dermis along with interstitial histiocytes and lymphocytes. **B.** Granuloma annulare-like pattern showing interstitial macrophages admixed with some neutrophils.

Leukocytoclastic Vasculitis

Leukocytoclastic vasculitis (LCV) represents a vascular reaction that is often idiopathic, but may be related to infections (fungal, gonococcal, meningococcal, rickettsial, leprosy, etc.), medications, immune complex mediated vasculitis (Henoch-Schönlein purpura, cryoglobulinemia, etc.), ANCA associated vasculitis (Wegener granulomatosis), connective tissue diseases, etc. The most characteristic clinical manifestation is palpable purpura, i.e., non-blanching erythematous papules, usually located in the lower extremities (183, 184).

HISTOLOGY (FIGURE 4-27A, B):
- Post capillary venules and capillary loops are primarily affected (often seen in superficial dermis).
- Endothelial cell swelling, fibrin deposition in the perivascular region, extravasation of red blood cells, and fragmentation of neutrophil nuclei (leukocytoclasis)
- Intravascular thrombi, ischemic necrosis of the epidermis, and subepidermal vesiculation
- Intraepidermal or subepidermal pustules
- **Note:** When noticing numerous eosinophils suspect a drug reaction or urticarial vasculitis.

DIFFERENTIAL DIAGNOSIS:
- LCV is a reaction pattern due to circulating immune complexes that can be secondary to a myriad of underlying disorders.

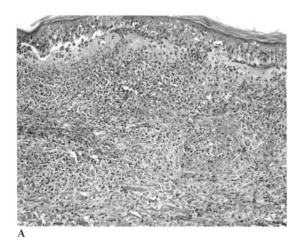 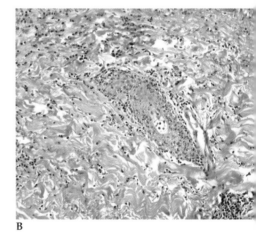

A   B

FIGURE 4-27 *Leukocytoclastic Vasculitis (LCV)*
A. Vessels in dermis showing fibrin deposition in the perivascular region, extravasation of red blood cells and neutrophils with leukocytoclasis. **B.** Higher magnification showing fibrin deposition in the perivascular region along with leukocytoclasia.

Granuloma Faciale

Granuloma faciale (GF) is an uncommon localized form of vasculitis of unknown etiology characterized by single or multiple cutaneous reddish brown nodules, usually occurring over the face of older patients. Male predilection has been observed (185).

HISTOLOGY (FIGURE 4-28):
- Dense polymorphic infiltrate in dermis composed of neutrophils (often with nuclear dust), eosinophils, lymphocytes, and plasma cells (often located in mid dermis but occasionally can involve the deep dermis and subcutaneous tissue)
- Extravasated red blood cells
- A "grenz" zone characteristically spares the papillary dermis between the inflammatory infiltrate and the overlying epidermis.
- Blood vessels appear dilated (ectatic) and can show leukocytoclastic vasculitis.
- In older lesions, fibrosis appears, and the density of the inflammatory infiltrate diminishes.

DIFFERENTIAL DIAGNOSIS:
- Erythema elevatum diutinum (EED) often shows more neutrophils, more sclerosis, and fewer numbers of eosinophils and plasma cells when compared to GF. See also EED.

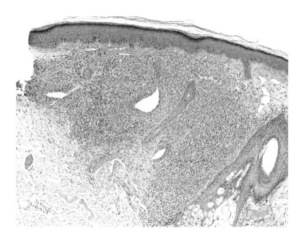

FIGURE 4-28 *Granuloma Faciale (GF)*
Dense neutrophilic infiltrate in upper half of dermis with a clear grenz zone and ectatic vessels.

Erythema Elevatum Diutinum

Erythema elevatum diutinum (EED), like GF, is a rare localized form of vasculitis. Papules, plaques, and nodules tend to cluster over joints, particularly the extensor surfaces of the hands, elbows, and ankles. EED has been described in association with a number of different clinical disorders including lymphoproliferative disorders, inflammatory bowel disease, rheumatoid arthritis, HIV, and SLE. An association with paraproteinemia is frequently present, often the IgA subtype (186, 187).

HISTOLOGY (FIGURE 4-29A, B):
- In early lesions, the presence of neutrophils in dermis with LCV is characteristic.
- In older lesions, the neutrophilic infiltrate declines and lesions develop fibrous scarring, sometimes giving a storiform ("plywood") appearance. Characteristic vertical oriented vessels. There may be only focal neutrophilic vasculitis.

DIFFERENTIAL DIAGNOSIS:
- Fully developed lesions can be indistinguishable from Sweet syndrome, neutrophilic drug reactions, Behcet syndrome, etc.
- EED is very similar to GF and the presence of increased number of eosinophils favors GF. Some authors have suggested a concept of vascular diseases that encompass GF and EED, regardless of the anatomic location.

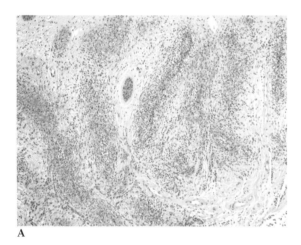 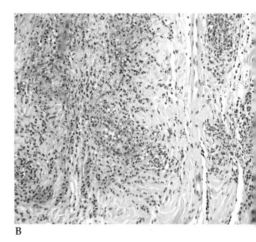

A   B

FIGURE 4-29 *Erythema Elevatum Diutinum (EED)*
A. The biopsy shows leukocytoclastic vasculitis, characterized by vascular destruction, hemorrhage, and a peri- and intravascular infiltrate of neutrophils with karyorrhexis. In addition, there is concentric vascular fibrosis. **B.** Higher magnification showing fibrinoid vascular necrosis, extravasation of erythrocytes, and an infiltrate of neutrophils displaying karyorrhexis.

Polyarteritis Nodosa

Polyarteritis nodosa (PN) is a systemic necrotizing vasculitis of small and medium-sized arteries. In addition to skin lesions, patients frequently present with multisystemic symptoms. Cutaneous involvement is seen in about 40% of patients, including purpura, cutaneous infarcts, livedo reticularis, and Reynaud phenomenon. Renal involvement, which is present in 75% of patients, is the most frequent cause of death. Microscopic polyangiitis (MPA) is a systemic pauci-immune necrotizing vasculitis that affects mainly small vessels. Cutaneous involvement in MPA is more common than in classic PN, and MPA is usually associated with antineutrophil cytoplasmic antibodies (ANCA) that are specific for myeloperoxidase (MPO) (188).

HISTOLOGY (FIGURE 4-30):
- PN is characterized by a necrotizing vasculitis (small and medium sized) seen mainly in deep dermis and subcutaneous fat.
- MPA is characterized by vasculitis of arteriole- and capillary-sized vessels.

DIFFERENTIAL DIAGNOSIS:
- The absence of involvement of capillaries and venules in PN is a major point of distinction with MPA; however, many vasculitic disorders show similar histologic features, especially in cases with only small vessel involvement, therefore, the biopsy findings should be correlated with the clinical information to determine the correct diagnosis.

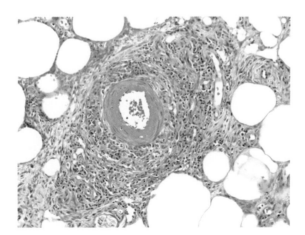

FIGURE 4-30 *Polyarteritis Nodosa (PN)*
Necrotizing vasculitis of a medium sized vessel in subcutaneous fat.

Churg-Strauss Syndrome (Allergic Granulomatosis)

Churg-Strauss syndrome (CSS) is characterized by asthma, allergic rhinitis, transient pulmonary infiltrates, and tissue and blood eosinophilia. CSS may show clinical and pathologic overlap with PN and Wegener granulomatosis. Like MPA, CSS has been associated with ANCA directed against myeloperoxidase (P-ANCA). Skin lesions are seen in 40%–70% of patients and include erythematous macules, hemorrhagic lesions ranging from petechiae to extensive ecchymoses, cutaneous and subcutaneous nodules, facial edema, livedo reticularis, and urticaria (189, 190).

HISTOLOGY (FIGURE 4-31):
- Necrotizing vasculitis
- Dense eosinophilic infiltrate
- A common feature is the "Churg-Strauss granuloma," i.e., degenerated collagen bundles surrounded by palisading histiocytes and multinucleated giant cells

DIFFERENTIAL DIAGNOSIS:
- The histologic features encountered in CSS are not entirely specific, so careful clinicopathological and serological evaluation is necessary to establish a definitive diagnosis.

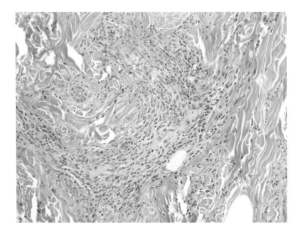

FIGURE 4-31 *Churg-Strauss Syndrome*
The biopsy shows a medium-sized vasculitis with eosinophilia.

Wegener Granulomatosis

Wegener granulomatosis (WG) is characterized by necrotizing granulomatous vasculitis of the upper and lower respiratory tracts, migratory/poliarticular arthralgia, glomerulonephritis, and a variable degree of small-vessel vasculitis. The majority of patients with WG have positive c-ANCA, which reacts with proteinase 3. Skin lesions occur in 14%–50% of patients and include palpable purpura and subcutaneous nodules with necrosis and ulceration that may be extensive. WG has a high mortality rate (191–193).

HISTOLOGY (FIGURE 4-32A,B):
- Leukocytoclastic vasculitis of small- to medium-sized vessels (fibrinoid necrosis, neutrophilic infiltrate, and karyorrhexis). Frankly granulomatous vasculitis is a rare feature.
- Extravasated red blood cells are invariably present.
- Geographic necrosis associated with mixed inflammatory response (histiocytes, giant cells, eosinophils, lymphocytes, and plasma cells).
- Occasional epidermal necrosis.
- Granulomatous inflammation in dermis, mimicking Churg-Strauss granuloma.
- In some cases only a perivascular lymphocytic infiltrate.

DIFFERENTIAL DIAGNOSIS:
- WG can show granulomatous inflammation in dermis, thus, mimicking sarcoidosis and infections (fungal and mycobacterial). WG can be easily confused with other forms of granulomatous/leukocytoclastic vasculitis. The presence of many eosinophils will favor the diagnosis of CSS over WG.

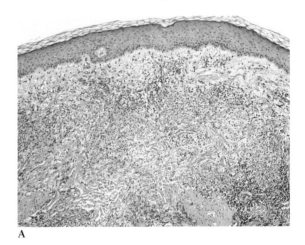 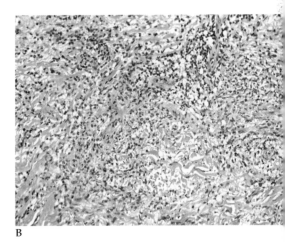

A   B

FIGURE 4-32 *Wegener Granulomatosis*
A. The biopsy shows small and medium-sized vessels surrounded by an infiltrate composed predominantly of epithelioid histiocytes, but also containing lymphocytes, neutrophils, and eosinophils. **B.** Higher magnification shows vasculitis characterized by an infiltrate composed predominantly of mononuclear cells but also containing small numbers of neutrophils.

Pigmented Purpuric Dermatosis (Capillaritis)

Pigmented purpuric dermatoses (PPD) are a group of chronic diseases of mostly unknown etiology that have a very distinctive clinical appearance. A number of clinical patterns of PPD are recognized that may represent different presentations of the same disorder. The term PPD includes Schamberg disease, purpura annularis telangiectodes (Majocchi disease), lichen aureus, eczematoid-like purpura of Doucas and Kapetanakis, pigmented purpuric lichenoid dermatosis of Gougerot and Blum, and itching purpura. There have been some cases of PPD progressing to mycosis fungoides (194, 195).

HISTOLOGY (FIGURE 4-33A, B):
- Variable extravasation of red blood cells in superficial dermis
- Hemosiderin laden macrophages in superficial dermis
- Variable infiltrate of lymphocytes in superficial dermis
- Few PMNs, especially in itching purpura
- Epidermis is usually normal or with mild spongiosis, exocytosis, and vacuolar damage.
- **Gougerot-Blum Variant:** often associated with a lichenoid lymphocytic infiltrate
- **Lichen Aureus:** a dense lymphohistiocytic infiltrate in upper dermis (band-like fashion)

DIFFERENTIAL DIAGNOSIS:
- Other vascular processes (old LCV, stasis dermatitis) can also result in extravasated red blood cells in the superficial dermis.
- PPD is usually located to a discrete anatomic area in contrast with LCV that usually involves large body areas.
- Stasis dermatitis is associated with clusters of thick-walled vessels. PPD cases with cytologic atypia of lymphocytes should be studied to rule out mycosis fungoides.

Pigmented Purpuric Dermatosis
(Capillaritis)

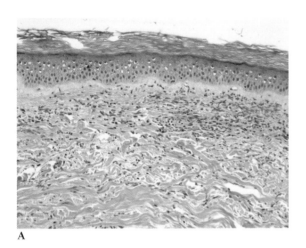

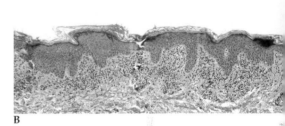

A

B

FIGURE 4-33 *Pigmented Purpuric Dermatoses (PPD)*
A. Schamberg disease showing extravasated red blood cells in superficial dermis.
B. Lichen aureus showing a lichenoid lymphohistiocytic infiltrate in superficial dermis and focal areas with extravasated red blood cells.

Cryoglobulinemia

Cryoglobulinemia is characterized by the presence of cryoglobulins in the serum. This may result in deposits of cryoglobulin-containing immune complexes, most commonly affecting the kidneys and skin. Type I cryoglobulinemia is the result of a monoclonal immunoglobulin (most commonly IgM), usually associated with an underlying lymphoma, myeloma, Waldestron macroglobulinemia, etc. Types II and III cryoglobulinemia (mixed and polyclonal cryoglobulinemia) contain rheumatoid factors (RFs), which are usually IgM, and are associated with connective tissue disease or infections such as Hepatitis C (196, 197).

HISTOLOGY (FIGURE 4-34A, B):
- **Type I Cryoglobulinemia:**
  - Vascular dilatation with endothelial swelling
  - Plugging of the vascular lumina by hyaline material (PAS positive)
  - Rarely, it can be associated with LCV
- **Type II and III Cryoglobulinemia:**
  - Leukocytoclastic vasculitis (LCV)

DIFFERENTIAL DIAGNOSIS:
- The differential diagnosis of Type I cryoglobulinemia is with other causes of thrombotic vasculopathy such as warfarin necrosis, protein C deficiency, etc.
- The differential diagnosis of Type II and III cryoglobulinemia is with other causes of LCV.

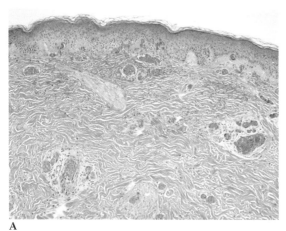 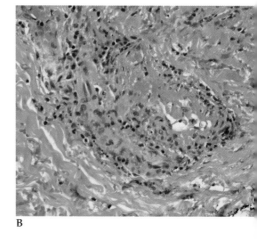

A   B

FIGURE 4-34 *Cryoglobulinemia*
A. Type I cryoglobulinemia showing dilated vascular spaces filled with hyaline material in a thrombus-like appearance. **B.** Type II cryoglobulinemia. The biopsy shows leukocytoclastic vasculitis.

Degos Disease
(Malignant Atrophic Papulosis)

Degos disease is an occlusive and progressive arteriopathy of small- and medium-size arteries, leading to tissue infarction and initially involving the skin. Clinically, it manifests initially with erythematous papules that when they heal leave scars with characteristic, central, porcelain white atrophic center. Degos disease occurs both in a limited benign cutaneous form and in a potentially lethal, multiorgan, systemic variant. In the latter variant, the gastrointestinal tract is affected in 50% of cases. Intestinal perforation is the most severe complication and the most common cause of death. Systemic manifestations usually develop from weeks to years after the onset of skin lesions, or, in rare instances, they may precede the skin lesions. Because of the broad overlap in clinical and histological findings, many authors have proposed that it may not be a specific entity but, rather, may represent a common end point to a variety of vascular insults (198).

HISTOLOGY:
- Hyperkeratotic and atrophic epidermis
- Wedge-shaped dermal infarction with broad base toward epidermis
- Mucin deposition
- Necrosis, edema, and sclerosis
- Vessels in deep dermis may show thrombosis, endothelial swelling, and a subtle perivascular lymphocytic infiltrate

DIFFERENTIAL DIAGNOSIS:
- Although the cutaneous findings of Degos disease are quite distinctive, similar lesions have been observed in patients with systemic diseases such as lupus and Crohn disease.

Atrophie Blanche
(Livedoid Vasculitis)

Atrophie blanche is usually seen in the lower legs of middle-aged or elderly females. Clinically, the lesions begin with purpuric papules and plaques and, ultimately, leave white, atrophic, stellate scars after the ulcers heal. There is an increased incidence during the winter and summer months. Platelet, coagulation, and fibrinolytic disorders have been reported in some cases of livedoid vasculitis, including lupus anticoagulant, protein C deficiency, and factor V mutation (Leiden). These may result in blood clots in the small vessels of the lower legs (199).

HISTOLOGY (FIGURE 4-35):
- Increased number of dermal vessels containing fibrin in vessel walls.
- Intraluminal fibrinoid plugs (PAS positive).
- Extravasated red blood cells and sparse lymphocytic inflammation.
- Infarct with hemorrhage can be seen in early lesions.
- Frank vasculitis is not a feature.
- The epidermis may be atrophic and dermis sclerotic (especially in late lesions).
- **DIF:** Perilesional skin shows deposits of immunoglobulins and complement in dermal blood vessels.

DIFFERENTIAL DIAGNOSIS:
- Stasis dermatitis may show some features observed in atrophie blanche; however, stasis dermatitis does not show the fibrinoid changes within the vessel wall.

Atrophie Blanche
(Livedoid Vasculitis)

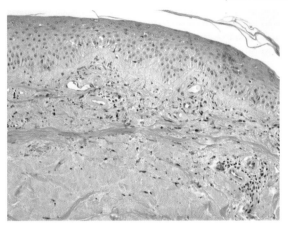

FIGURE 4-35 *Atrophie Blanche*
Fibrinoid material and thickening of vessel wall.

Calciphylaxis

Calciphylaxis is a rare dermatosis that is associated with calcification of small- and medium-sized vessels resulting in ischemic necrosis of the skin. It is characterized by exquisitely tender purpuric lesions, most often located on the medial thighs or buttocks. Calciphylaxis most often affects patients with end-stage renal disease (ESRD) undergoing hemodialysis or peritoneal dialysis and patients with kidney transplantation. Usually these patients have secondary hyperparathyroidism. The prognosis of this condition is extremely poor. Occasionally the diagnosis can be suspected when calcium deposits in the subcutaneous vessels are detected in MRIs (200, 201).

HISTOLOGY (FIGURE 4-36A, B):
- Calcification of small vessels in deep dermis and subcutaneous tissue
- Fibrin thrombi
- Sometimes intimal proliferation of small vessels with luminal narrowing
- Ischemic necrosis of skin and subcutaneous tissue is a frequent finding
- Rarely there is also foreign body reaction to the calcific deposits

DIFFERENTIAL DIAGNOSIS:
- Other dermatoses, such as metastatic calcifications, cutaneous calcinosis, gout, and pseudogout, may show extravascular calcium deposits but they lack the characteristic, prominent vascular involvement of calciphylaxis.
- Arteriosclerosis (Monckeberg disease) may also show calcification of the vessels, but the involved vessel is usually larger than the ones seen in calciphylaxis.

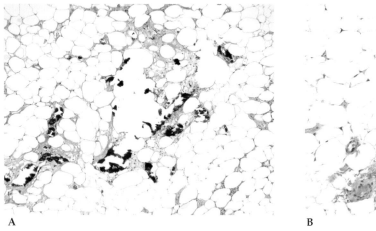 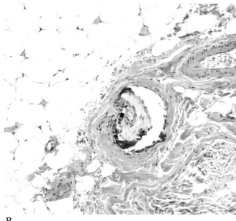

A   B

FIGURE 4-36 *Calciphylaxis*
A. Areas of calcification in subcutaneous fat. **B.** Calcification of small vessels in deep dermis.

Scurvy

Scurvy results from a deficiency of vitamin C (ascorbic acid). Clinically, the lesions characteristically have a perifollicular distribution, but there may also be spontaneous petechiae and ecchymoses. Other features include follicular hyperkeratosis, abnormal hair growth with the formation of corkscrew hairs, bleeding gums, and poor wound healing (202, 203).

HISTOLOGY (FIGURE 4-37):
- Perifollicular and perivascular extravasated red blood cells
- Follicular hyperkeratosis with coiled and fragmented hairs (corkscrew hair)

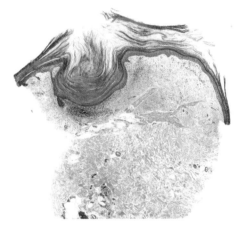

FIGURE 4-37 *Scurvy*
The biopsy shows a dilated, plugged follicle and immediately surrounding the follicle, there is some hemorrhage and an inflammatory infiltrate composed of lymphocytes, histiocytes, and neutrophils.

Morphea/Scleroderma

Morphea, also known as localized scleroderma, is a dermatosis characterized by thickening and induration of the skin and subcutaneous tissue due to excessive collagen deposition. Clinically, presents as a single plaque with a white center and erythematous border. Young to middle-aged women are most commonly affected, and no systemic disease is identified. Systemic scleroderma is a chronic multiorgan disease commonly affecting the kidneys, lungs, and gastrointestinal tract (esophageal dysmotility) in addition to the skin. The skin is indurated often with hypo or hyperpigmentation and commonly affects the trunk, extremities, face, and fingers. Systemic scleroderma is most commonly seen in young to middle-aged women (204–207).

HISTOLOGY (FIGURE 4-38A, B):
- Epidermis may be atrophic
- Thickened and sclerotic collagen bundles
- Collagen replaces the fat around the skin adnexa and extends into the subcutis.
- Atrophy of the pilosebaceous units
- Eccrine glands are located at a high level in dermis
- Subtle superficial and deep dermal lymphoplasmacytic infiltrate (occasionally eosinophils)
- Lymphocytic aggregates and plasma cells at the dermal–subcutaneous junction
- Thickening of the wall of small blood vessels and narrowing of their lumen

DIFFERENTIAL DIAGNOSIS:
- While morphea and systemic scleroderma share many histological features, the lesions of morphea are usually more inflammatory than in systemic scleroderma.

Morphea/Scleroderma

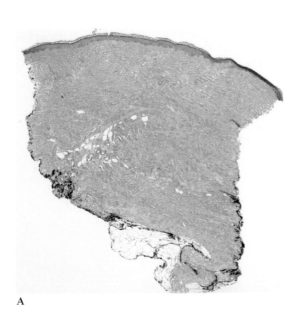

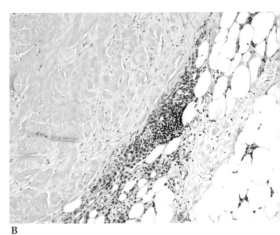

A

B

FIGURE 4-38 *Morphea*
A. Thickened and sclerotic collagen bundles in dermis replacing skin adnexa.
B. Characteristic lymphoplasmacytic infiltrate in dermal subcutaneous junction.

Nephrogenic Systemic Fibrosis

Nephrogenic systemic fibrosis (NSF), also known as nephrogenic fibrosing dermopathy (NFD), is a dermatosis that occurs in patients with renal insufficiency who have had imaging studies with gadolinium, a contrast agent used in imaging studies. Most patients have had treatments that include hemodialysis, peritoneal dialysis, or renal transplantation. Clinically, these patients present with scleroderma-like plaques often involving the extremities. There may also be distinct papules and subcutaneous nodules (208, 209).

HISTOLOGY (FIGURE 4-39A, B):
- Thickening of the collagen bundles in dermis
- Thickening of fibrous septa of the subcutis
- Proliferation of spindle cells (fibroblasts)
- Irregular distribution of elastic fibers
- Cleft-like spaces surrounding the thickened collagen bundles
- Common deposition of mucin in dermis
- Dermal stroma often shows multinucleated and large epithelioid and stellate cells
- Spindle cells (fibroblasts) are positive for CD34

DIFFERENTIAL DIAGNOSIS:
- NSF has histological overlap with scleromyxedema since both have thickened collagen bundles, fibroblasts, and mucin deposition; however, the presence of increased mucin and inflammatory infiltrate is a common feature of scleromyxedema. NSF involves the subcutis as opposed to scleromyxedema, which is usually limited to the dermis. If necessary, mass spectrophotometry may be used to detect the presence of gadolinium in tissue.

Nephrogenic Systemic Fibrosis

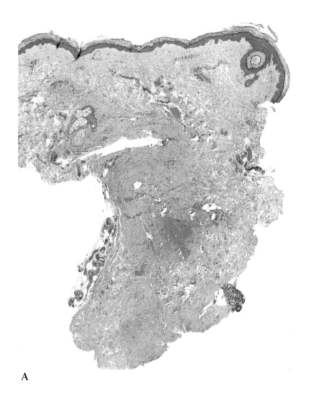

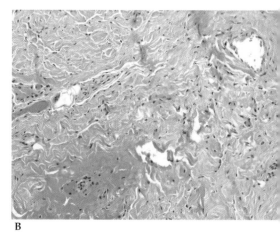

A

B

FIGURE 4-39 *Nephrogenic Systemic Fibrosis (NSF)*
A. Thickened collagen bundles in dermis with a subtle proliferation of spindle cell fibroblasts. **B.** Higher magnification showing the increased number of spindle cells with focal mucin deposition.

Radiation Dermatitis

Radiation dermatitis occurs in patients receiving radiotherapy, with or without chemo-therapy. In most patients, the radiation dermatitis is mild to moderate, but 20%-25% of patients experience severe reactions. There is a well-defined progression of changes following irradiation of the skin usually divided into early changes and chronic changes arising many months or years after the initial exposure. In the acute form, there is variable erythema and hair loss. The chronic form shows poikiloderma with atrophy, telangiectasias, pigmentary changes, and loss of appendages (210).

HISTOLOGY (FIGURE 4-40):
- **Acute Form:** Mild spongiosis, edema of papillary dermis, epidermal necrosis, vascular ectasia, and thrombosis
- **Subacute Form:** Usually shows a lichenoid tissue reaction with interface dermatitis and dyskeratotic keratinocytes.
- **Chronic Form:** The epidermal changes include epidermal atrophy, hyperkeratosis, mild basal vacuolar changes and dyskeratotic cells. The main changes are located in dermis and show dermal sclerosis and hyalinization, loss of adnexa, stellate fibro-blasts (bizarre fibroblasts), telangiectatic vessels in superficial dermis with hyalin-ization and thrombosis.

DIFFERENTIAL DIAGNOSIS:
- The chronic phase of radiation dermatitis will show changes indistinguishable from those seen in late stage of burns and morphea; however, the presence of bizarre fibroblasts will favor the diagnosis of radiation dermatitis.

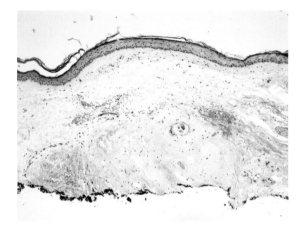

FIGURE 4-40 *Radiation Dermatitis*
Chronic phase showing atrophy of epidermis with dermal sclerosis, hyalinization and loss of adnexal structures.

Pseudoxanthoma Elasticum

Pseudoxanthoma elasticum (PXE) is a rare, genetic disorder characterized by calcification and fragmentation of elastic fibers in the skin, eyes (angioid streaks of retina), and the cardiovascular system. Mutations in the ABCC6 gene on chromosome 16p13.1 are responsible for this condition. Clinically, the lesions of PXE usually develop in early childhood and are noted in adolescence, with characteristic yellowish papules with a predilection for flexural creases, particularly in the neck. Acquired PXE refers to an etiologically and clinically diverse group of patients with late onset of the disease, no family history, absence of vascular and retinal changes, and identical histologic changes. Also patients on chronic penicillamine may show lesions reminiscent of PXE (211, 212).

HISTOLOGY (FIGURE 4-41):
■ Numerous wavy, fragmented, and basophilic granular elastic fibers in mid reticular dermis
■ The elastic fibers stain black with both Verhoeff elastic stain and Von Kossa stain.

DIFFERENTIAL DIAGNOSIS:
■ PXE-like fibers have been seen in other skin dermatoses such as lipodermatosclerosis, morphea, calciphylaxis, erythema nodosum, granuloma annulare, lichen sclerosus, etc. However, in those diseases the fibers are usually very small in number.

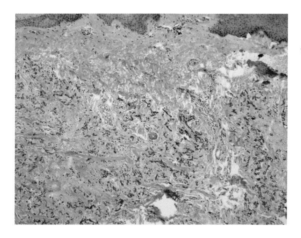

FIGURE 4-41 *Pseudoxanthoma Elasticum (PXE)* Numerous wavy, fragmented and basophilic elastic fibers in dermis.

Eosinophilic Fasciitis (Shulman Syndrome)

Eosinophilic fasciitis (EF) is a rare, localized fibrosing disorder of the fascia. Clinically, it presents by pain and symmetrical thickening of the dermis and subcutaneous tissue, often in a rope-like fashion. Onset follows strenuous exercise in 50% of the cases. Patients frequently have associated peripheral eosinophilia and hypergamma-globulinemia (213, 214).

HISTOLOGY (FIGURE 4-42):
- Deep dermal sclerosis and fibrosis of septa between fat lobules associated with an inflamed and thickened fascia
- Mixed inflammatory infiltrate composed of lymphocytes, plasma cells, and variable numbers of eosinophils

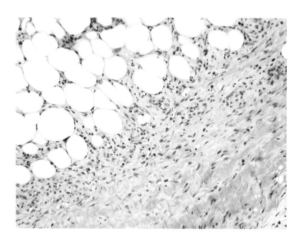

FIGURE 4-42 *Eosinophilic Fasciitis*
Deeper dermis sclerosis with increased number of eosinophils.

Connective Tissue Nevus

Connective tissue nevi are cutaneous hamartomas in which one of the components of the extracellular connective tissue is present in abnormal amounts. Collagenomas and elastomas are considered within this category. Collagenomas present as asymptomatic plaques and nodules on the trunk and upper part of the arms. They have been reported in the MEN type I syndrome. Familial connective tissue nevi may be seen as a solitary lesion or be associated with the Buschke–Ollendorff syndrome (osteopoikilosis). The Shagreen patch is a distinct variant of collagenoma, found almost exclusively in patients with tuberous sclerosis, and clinically presents as elevated, flesh-colored plaques on the trunk (215, 216).

HISTOLOGY:
- **Collagenoma:** Thickening of the dermis showing broad collagen bundles in a haphazard arrangement. Elastic fibers are widely spaced and sometimes are thin and fragmented. The epidermis is normal but occasionally there may be an epidermal nevus (**Figure 4-43**).
- **Shagreen Patch:** Reticular dermis shows dense sclerotic bundles of collagen with an interwoven pattern. Fibroblasts appear hypertrophied.
- Connective tissue nevi in the Buschke-Ollendorff syndrome more commonly are of the elastic tissue type (dermatofibrosis lenticularis disseminata). Histologically, they show a characteristic increase in elastic fibers that are broad and interlacing.

DIFFERENTIAL DIAGNOSIS:
- Collagenomas may be difficult to separate from morphea/scleroderma, which usually show a diffuse homogenization of collagen, inflammatory infiltrate and obliteration of adnexal structures.

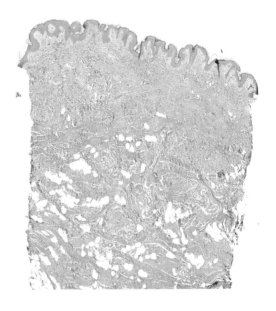

FIGURE 4-43 *Collagenoma*
Coarse collagen fibers, leading to dermal thickening.

Focal Dermal Hypoplasia
(Goltz Syndrome)

Focal dermal hypoplasia (Goltz syndrome) is a rare syndrome with multiple congenital malformations affecting particularly the skin, eyes, bones, and teeth, and inherited as an X-linked dominant trait, which is usually lethal in males. Cutaneous manifestations include widespread areas of dermal thinning in a reticular and linear pattern with soft yellowish nodules representing herniations of subcutaneous fat through an underdeveloped dermis (217, 218).

HISTOLOGY:
- Markedly thinned dermis with loose collagen bundles
- Superficial extension of adipocytes into superficial dermis

DIFFERENTIAL DIAGNOSIS:
- Nevus lipomatosus usually shows the presence of adipocytes in superficial dermis; however, it lacks the attenuation and loose collagen bundle seen in focal dermal hypoplasia.

Kyrle Disease
(Hyperkeratosis Follicularis et Parafollicularis in Cutem Penetrans)

Kyrle disease is a rare perforating dermatosis that is associated with patients with chronic renal failure, hemodialysis, and diabetes. Clinically, it is characterized by formation of large papules with central keratin plugs usually on the lower extremities but it may develop in a widespread distribution pattern (219, 220).

HISTOLOGY (FIGURE 4-44):
- Keratotic plug within an invaginated atrophic epidermis (bordered by marked epidermal acanthosis)
- Focal parakeratosis can be seen deep in the plug.
- Within the plug often there is some basophilic cellular debris.
- Surrounding mixed inflammatory infiltrate usually is present, including neutrophils, lymphocytes, and giant cells.
- Absence of elastic tissue

DIFFERENTIAL DIAGNOSIS:
- Elastosis perforans serpiginosa (EPS) and reactive perforating collagenosis (RPC) may look alike histologically; however, EPS shows degenerated elastic tissue while RPC contains collagen bundles.

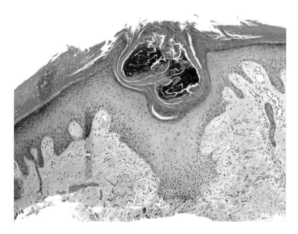

FIGURE 4-44 *Kyrle Disease*
The biopsy shows an epidermal invagination in the center of the specimen. It is filled with keratotic and parakeratotic material, basophilic debris, and inflammatory cells.

Elastosis Perforans Serpiginosa

Elastosis perforans serpiginosa (EPS) is a rare skin dermatosis in which abnormal elastic tissue fibers and cellular debris are expelled from the papillary dermis through the epidermis (transepithelial elimination). EPS occurs in three forms: Idiopathic, reactive (associated with Down syndrome, Ehlers-Danlos syndrome, Marfan syndrome, diabetes, renal failure, scleroderma, PXE, etc.), and drug-induced (caused by D-penicillamine) (221).

HISTOLOGY (FIGURE 4-45):
- Narrow transepidermal channel with basophilic nuclear debris and brightly eosinophilic fragmented "elastic" fibers
- The transepidermal channel is bordered by acanthotic and hyperkeratotic epidermis.
- Keratinocytic plug may overlie the channel.
- Verhoeff-Van Gieson stain shows increased numbers of coarse elastic fibers in the papillary dermis. (Note: In penicillamine-induced EPS the elastic fibers appear irregular, sawtoothed, and serrated).

DIFFERENTIAL DIAGNOSIS:
- See above

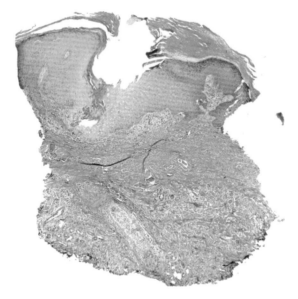

FIGURE 4-45 *Elastosis Perforans Serpiginosa (EPS)*
Transepidermal channel with keratotic plug and focal basophilic nuclear debris.

Perforating Folliculitis

Perforating folliculitis (PF) is an asymptomatic dermatosis in which keratotic follicular papules develop particularly over the extensor surfaces. It may present as an isolated finding but can also be associated with chronic renal failure and diabetes mellitus. Kyrle disease may simply represent an exaggerated form of perforating folliculitis (222, 223).

HISTOLOGY (FIGURE 4-46):
- Dilated hair follicle with ortho and parakeratotic keratin
- The infundibular follicular epithelium is disrupted (single or multiple foci).
- Connective-tissue elements, including collagen and elastin, and varying numbers of inflammatory cells can be found within this transfollicular channel and within the follicular lumen.
- Curled-up hair can be seen within the keratinous plug and/or within the transfollicular channel.

DIFFERENTIAL DIAGNOSIS:
- The main differential diagnosis is with Kyrle disease. PF usually shows a symmetric follicular involvement associated with infundibular epithelial perforation, as opposed in Kyrle disease where the perforation is at the base. EPS usually shows more elastic fibers when compared with PF.

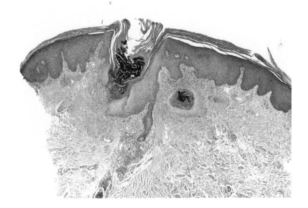

FIGURE 4-46 *Perforating Folliculitis*
The biopsy shows a dilated, hyperkeratotic, follicular infundibulum filled with orthokeratotic and parakeratotic material, necrotic debris, and degenerated inflammatory cells. A perforation is apparent near the base of the infundibulum. Degenerated connective tissue fibrosis appear to be entering the infundibulum through this perforation.

Reactive Perforating Collagenosis

Reactive perforating collagenosis (RPC) is a rare skin disorder characterized by the transepidermal elimination of altered collagen through the epidermis. There are two distinct clinical forms, the inherited form that manifests in childhood and an acquired sporadic form that occurs in adulthood (associated with diabetes, chronic renal failure, and malignancy) (220, 224).

HISTOLOGY:
- In established lesions, a cup-shaped depression of the epidermis which is filled with a keratin plug containing parakeratosis, inflammatory debris, and collagen fibers.
- Vertically orientated basophilic collagen fibers are seen in the underlying dermis with focal extrusion through the epidermis.
- Absence of elastic fibers
- The epidermis is usually atrophic and may show ulceration; however, at the edges of the cup-shaped invagination the epidermis is acanthotic.
- Occasional follicular involvement

DIFFERENTIAL DIAGNOSIS:
- See above

Inflammatory Reactions Primarily Involving the Subcutaneous Tissue

5

Erythema Nodosum

Erythema nodosum (EN) is an acute inflammatory condition that presents with symmetrical, tender, erythematous nodules and raised plaques usually limited to the anterior aspects of the lower legs. EN is presumed to be a hypersensitivity reaction and may occur in association with several systemic diseases including infections (streptococcal infection are the most common etiology in children), sarcoidosis, rheumatologic diseases, inflammatory bowel diseases, medications, Sweet syndrome, autoimmune disorders and malignancies (225–227).

HISTOLOGY (FIGURE 5-1A–C):
- Septal panniculitis with small foci of inflammatory cells extending into the adjacent lobular fat
- Thickening of the septa
- Only peripheral involvement of the fat lobules (center of the lobule is spared; however, in chronic lesions the complete lobule may be affected)
- The septal infiltrate is predominantly lymphocytic, but it may contain variable numbers of giant cells (foreign body type), few eosinophils and histiocytes
- Nodular aggregates of epithelioid histiocytes arranged around a cleft-like space (Miescher granuloma)
- Endothelial swelling of small septal vessels; sometimes a lymphocytic cuffing of septal venules
- Rarely, definite vasculitis
- Early lesions are characterized by septal inflammation (mainly composed of neutrophils), edema, and hemorrhage within the septa
- In older lesions, marked septal fibrosis

DIFFERENTIAL DIAGNOSIS:
- The differential diagnosis of this condition is broad since several dermatoses in their acute phase may show septal panniculitis (infections, connective tissue diseases, vasculitis, trauma, etc.). Special stains and careful clinical evaluation will help in the differential diagnosis.

Erythema Nodosum

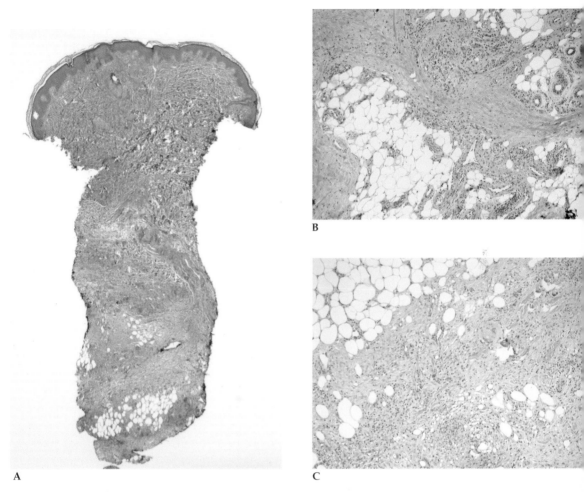

A   C

FIGURE 5-1 *Erythema Nodosum (EN)*
A. Septal panniculitis with perilobular granulomatous inflammation and septal fibrosis. **B.** Higher magnification showing the septae with fibrosis and sparse chronic inflammatory response. **C.** Nodular aggregates of epithelioid histiocytes around fat lobules (Miescher granulomas).

Pancreatic Panniculitis

Pancreatic panniculitis is usually manifested by multiple, purple, painful erythematous nodules. Lesions are tender and may occur at any site but show a predilection for the lower extremities, buttocks, and trunk. The lesions are associated with acute pancreatitis or pancreatic neoplasms (228, 229).

HISTOLOGY (FIGURE 5-2):
- Lobular panniculitis with histiocytes and lymphocytes
- Enzymatic fat necrosis in a pattern similar to that observed in the peripancreatic abdominal adipose tissue after pancreatic damage
- Granular basophilic degeneration of fat results in "ghost cells"
- Calcification specially at the periphery of necrotic zones
- Neutrophilic infiltration is usually seen around the foci of fat necrosis and the uninvolved fat is heavily infiltrated by acute and chronic infiltrate

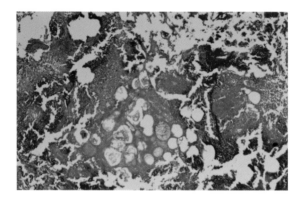

FIGURE 5-2 *Pancreatic Panniculitis*
Enzymatic fat necrosis, with granular basophilic degeneration of fat resulting in "ghost cells."

Alpha-1-Antitrypsin Deficiency

Aplha-1-antitrypsin deficiency is a genetic disorder characterized by low serum levels of alpha-1-antitrypsin resulting in recurrent ulcerated panniculitis. The gene (PI) encoding this protease inhibitor is situated at 14q32.1. Clinically, patients present with recurrent subcutaneous nodules that involves the extremities, buttocks, face, and trunk. Patients often have other manifestation of the disease including emphysema, hepatitis, and acquired angioedema (230, 231).

HISTOLOGY (FIGURE 5-3):
■ The panniculitis can be lobular and septal.
■ **Lobular Panniculitis:** Characterized by neutrophilic inflammation and necrosis of fat lobules.
■ **Septal Panniculitis:** Also shows neutrophilic and histiocytic inflammation but of the fibrous septa along with liquefactive necrosis of the dermis.

DIFFERENTIAL DIAGNOSIS:
■ The lobular pattern of alpha-1-antitrypsin is indistinguishable from other forms of lobular panniculitis, especially lobular panniculitis secondary from infections or factitial agents.

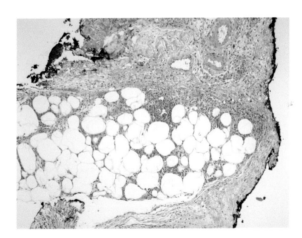

FIGURE 5-3 *Alpha-1-Antitrypsin Deficiency*
Septal and lobular panniculitis with increased number of neutrophils.

Erythema Induratum (Nodular Vasculitis)

Erythema induratum and nodular vasculitis have been considered by many authors the same disease for a long time. Some authors have proposed an erythema induratum/nodular vasculitis complex with two variants: erythema induratum of Bazin type (associated with tuberculosis) and nodular vasculitis or erythema induratum of Whitfield-type (non-TBC). Clinically, they both are characterized by recurrent crops of tender erythematous nodules, usually with a predilection for the calves, although the shins can be involved (232, 233).

HISTOLOGY (FIGURE 5-4A, B):
- Mixed or lobular granulomatous panniculitis with vasculitis.
- The inflammatory infiltrate is mixed containing lymphocytes, scattered neutrophils, and macrophages.
- There are also tuberculoid-type granulomas with foreign body– and Langhans-type giant cells (granulomas may show caseation which may be then associated with tuberculosis).
- Vasculitis involves both arteries and veins, ranging from small to medium-sized vessels, occasional necrotizing vasculitis (vasculitis not always identified).

DIFFERENTIAL DIAGNOSIS:
- Special stains are needed to rule out an infectious etiology.
- Sarcoidosis also enters in the differential diagnosis; however, granulomas in sarcoidosis are located higher in dermis.

Erythema Induratum
(Nodular Vasculitis)

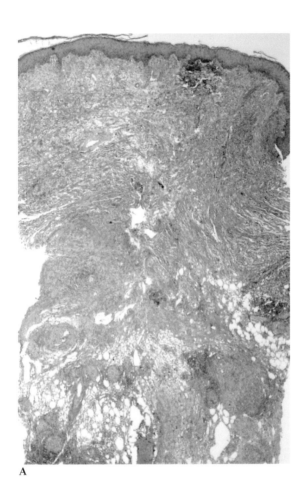

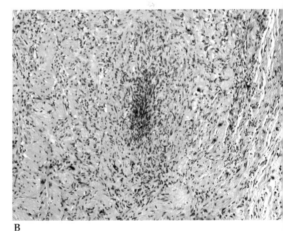

A

B

FIGURE 5-4 *Erythema Induratum*
A. Mixed granulomatous panniculitis with non-caseating granulomas. **B.** Higher magnification showing medium-sized vessel granulomatous vasculitis.

Subcutaneous Fat Necrosis of the Newborn

Subcutaneous fat necrosis of the newborn (SCFN) is an uncommon disorder that generally occurs in full-term healthy neonates in the first several weeks of life. Clinically, SCFN develop plaques and nodules that tend to be distributed over bone prominences, including cheeks, shoulders, back, buttocks, and thighs and usually runs a self-limited course, but it may be complicated by hypercalcemia and other metabolic abnormalities. The pathogenesis of SCFN is not well understood but some cases have been related to some degree of fetal distress (232, 234).

HISTOLOGY (FIGURE 5-5A, B):
- Lobular panniculitis associated with a mixed inflammatory infiltrate composed of lymphocytes, neutrophils, histiocytes, and multinucleated giant cells (rare eosinophils).
- Both adipocytes and giant cells contain the characteristic needle-shaped clefts that represent dissolved fat crystals.
- Calcification of interlobular septa along with fibrosis may also be a feature in older lesions.
- Focal fat necrosis is present and this may lead to fat cyst formation.

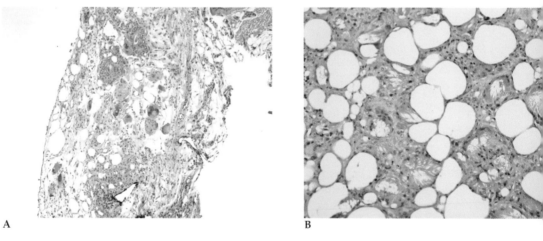

A   B

FIGURE 5-5 *Subcutaneous Fat Necrosis of the Newborn*
A. Lobular panniculitis with many multinucleated giant cells. **B.** Both adipocytes and giant cells contain the characteristic needle-shaped clefts that represent dissolved fat crystals.

Sclerema Neonatorum

Sclerema neonatorum is a rare disease associated with high morbidity and mortality that is characterized clinically by diffuse thickening and induration of a large percentage of the body surface. Palms, soles, and scrotum are characteristically spared. In contrast to SCFN, sclerema neonatorum is a crystalline panniculitis associated with serious neonatal illness. Neonates with sclerema neonatorum are frequently premature and commonly have other illnesses, such as infection and dehydration (232).

HISTOLOGY (FIGURE 5-6):
■ Lipocytes with needle-shaped clefts radially oriented (starburst pattern)
■ Rare giant cells
■ Minimal inflammation
■ No to mild fat necrosis
■ Subcutaneous septa are often widened by edema

DIFFERENTIAL DIAGNOSIS:
■ SCFN differs from sclerema neonatorum by showing radial clefts predominantly in macrophages, fat necrosis, and greater degree of inflammation.

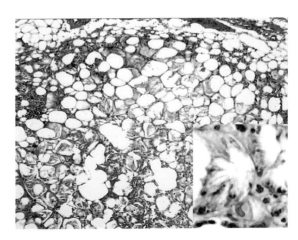

FIGURE 5-6 *Sclerema Neonatorum*
Primarily lipocytes showing the characteristic needle-shaped clefts radially oriented in a starburst pattern.

Lupus Erythematosus Profundus (Lupus Panniculitis)

Lupus erythematosus profundus is a rare variant of panniculitis that represents a complication in approximately 1–3% of patients with cutaneous lupus erythematosus (systemic and discoid forms). Most commonly it occurs in adult women and presents as multiple nodules or plaques on the proximal extremities, lower back and trunk. Patients usually experience recurrent lesions that resolve, leaving areas of lipoatrophy and scarring (235–237).

HISTOLOGY (FIGURE 5-7A–C):
- Lobular panniculitis associated with lymphocytic infiltrate (lobular lymphocytic panniculitis)
- Hyaline necrosis of fat lobules, karyorrhexis, and a lymphoplasmacytic infiltrate (eosinophils can be seen in up 25% of cases)
- Characteristically, the subcutaneous tissue contains lymphoid follicles with germinal centers adjacent to fibrous septa (20–50% of cases)
- Blood vessels may demonstrate "onion-skin" thickening and a lymphocytic vasculitis possibly with lymphocytic nuclear dust
- Lymphocytic infiltrate around the perineural sheath
- Epidermal and dermal changes of lupus erythematosus in up to 50% of cases (interface damage, superficial and deep perivascular lymphocytic infiltrate with perifollicular involvement and dermal mucin deposition)

DIFFERENTIAL DIAGNOSIS:
- The main differential diagnosis of this entity is with subcutaneous panniculitis-like T-cell lymphoma (SPTCL). The most useful criteria for distinguishing lupus erythematosus profundus from SPTCL are the presence of epidermal and dermal changes seen in lupus (interface damage and mucin deposition). Lymphoid follicles are uncommon in other panniculitides but they are occasionally seen in morphea, erythema nodosum, and erythema induratum.

Lupus Erythematosus Profundus
(Lupus Panniculitis)

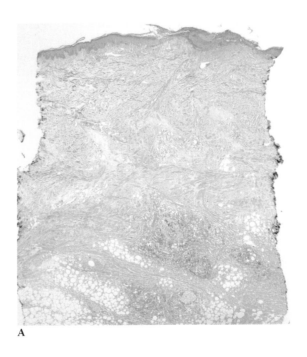

A

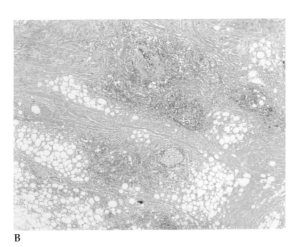

B

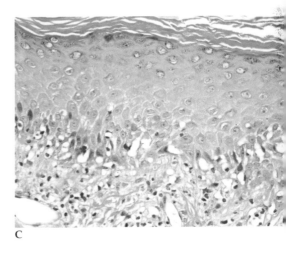

C

FIGURE 5-7 *Lupus Profundus*
A. Lobular panniculitis with prominent lymphocytic infiltrate. Many lymphoid follicles with germinal center formation are noted. **B.** Higher magnification showing the reactive lymphoid follicles. **C.** The overlying epidermis showing focal interface vacuolar damage of the dermal epidermal junction.

Lipodermatosclerosis (Sclerosing Panniculitis)

Lipodermatosclerosis is uncommon and it is associated with venous or arterial insufficiency. It presents as tender, indurated bilateral plaques in the lower legs. Lipomembranous panniculitis is a form of fat necrosis associated not only with stasis, but also with autoimmune disease, peripheral vascular disease, and infections (232, 238, 239).

HISTOLOGY (FIGURE 5-8A, B):
- In early stages, lobular and septal panniculitis with lymphocytic infiltrate along with vascular thrombosis
- Hyalinization of fat lobule with microcysts (amorphous eosinophilic material lining microcysts in arabesque pattern)
- Membranous fat necrosis
- Septal scarring and sclerosis (sometimes atrophy of the subcutaneous fat)
- Stasis changes are commonly seen in dermis (fibrosis, lobular capillary proliferation, thickening of vessel wall, fibrosis, hemosiderin deposition)

DIFFERENTIAL DIAGNOSIS:
- The end stage of lipodermatosclerosis may show a sclerodermoid reaction mimicking morphea and/or scleroderma; however, the presence of stasis changes will help to establish the correct diagnosis.

Lipodermatosclerosis
(Sclerosing Panniculitis)

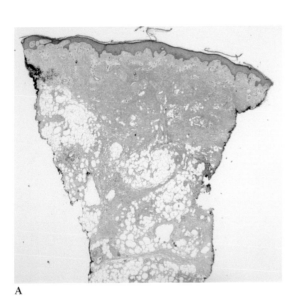

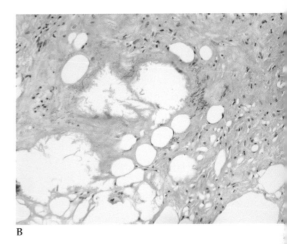

A

B

FIGURE 5-8 *Lipodermatosclerosis*
A. Lobular and septal panniculitis with hyalinization of the fat lobule. **B.** Hyalinization
of fat lobule with microcysts showing the amorphous eosinophilic material lining
microcysts in arabesque pattern.

Cutaneous Deposition and Metabolic Disorders

6

LOCALIZED PRETIBIAL MYXEDEMA (THYROID DERMOPATHY)

LICHEN MYXEDEMATOSUS (PAPULAR MUCINOSIS)/ SCLEROMYXEDEMA

SCLEREDEMA

RETICULAR ERYTHEMATOUS MUCINOSIS

DIGITAL MUCOUS CYST

MUCOCELE

FOCAL DERMAL MUCINOSIS

AMYLOIDOSIS

COLLOID MILIUM

LIPOID PROTEINOSIS

XANTHOMATOSIS

GOUT

CALCINOSIS CUTIS

OCHRONOSIS

ARGYRIA (SILVER DEPOSITION)

LOCALIZED PRETIBIAL MYXEDEMA (THYROID DERMOPATHY)

Pretibial myxedema is a term used to describe localized lesions that result from the deposition of hyaluronic acid. Clinically, pretibial myxedema presents as nodular lesions with elephantiasis-like thickening of the skin. The anterior aspect of the lower legs, sometimes with spread to the dorsum of the feet, is the most common site of involvement, although the upper trunk, upper extremities, and even the face, neck or ears have been rarely involved. It is nearly always associated with Graves disease (seen in 1%–4% of cases and always associated with exophthalmos); however, it may also occur in patients with non-thyrotoxic Graves disease and occasionally in association with Hashimoto thyroiditis (240).

HISTOLOGY (FIGURE 6-1A, B):

- Deposition of mucin throughout the reticular dermis (mid and lower dermis).
- Mucin may appear as individual threads and granules with wide separation of collagen bundles.
- Attenuation of collagen fibers.
- There is no increase in fibroblasts (occasionally few stellate single fibroblasts).
- Mild superficial perivascular lymphocytic infiltrate.
- The overlying epidermis may show hyperkeratosis (sometimes follicular plugging).
- Alcian-blue (pH of 2.5) and colloidal iron stains highlight the hyaluronic acid mucin.

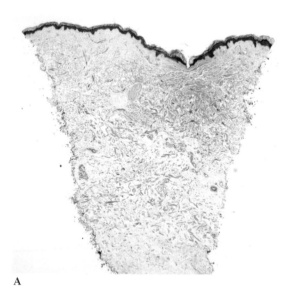
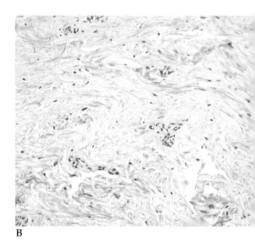

A   B

FIGURE 6-1 *Pretibial Myxedema*
A. Mucin deposition throughout reticular dermis. **B.** Higher magnification showing mucin deposition with very few single fibroblasts.

LICHEN MYXEDEMATOSUS (PAPULAR MUCINOSIS)/ SCLEROMYXEDEMA

The localized form is generally called lichen myxedematosus (papular mucinosis), and the more sclerotic, diffuse form is referred to as scleromyxedema. Lichen myxedematosus (papular mucinosis) presents with multiple pale papules that develop on the face, neck, hands, forearms, and trunk. Scleromyxedema presents with lichenoid papules and plaques that are accompanied by skin thickening involving almost the entire body (face, neck, forearms, and hands are sites of predilection). A paraproteinemia, usually IgG lambda, is almost always present in scleromyxedema and sometimes in papular mucinosis. Other associations are hepatitis C and HIV infection and ingestion of toxic oil (240, 241).

HISTOLOGY (FIGURE 6-2):
■ Deposits of mucin in dermis
■ Marked proliferation of plump stellate fibroblasts and increased collagen thickening in upper and mid dermis
■ The fibroblasts are irregularly arranged and the collagen may have a whorled pattern
■ Secondary changes such as flattening of the epidermis and atrophy of pilosebaceous follicles
■ Elastic fibers may be fragmented
■ Often sparse perivascular infiltrate of lymphocytes (sometimes with eosinophils and mast cells)
■ Alcian-blue (pH of 2.5) and colloidal iron stains highlight the hyaluronic acid mucin

DIFFERENTIAL DIAGNOSIS:
■ NSF has histological overlap with scleromyxedema since both have thickened collagen bundles, fibroblasts and mucin deposition; however, the presence of increased mucin and inflammatory infiltrate is a common feature of scleromyxedema. NSF involves the subcutis as opposed to scleromyxedema.

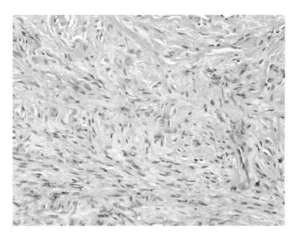

FIGURE 6-2 *Scleromyxedema*
Mucin deposition in dermis with a marked proliferation of plump stellate fibroblasts.

SCLEREDEMA

Clinically, scleredema is characterized by non-pitting induration of the skin with a predilection for the posterior neck, shoulders, upper trunk, and face. Scleredema can be categorized into three clinical subgroups: 1) After acute respiratory infection, particularly an upper respiratory tract streptococcal infection, 2) associated with a monoclonal gammopathy, and 3) associated with diabetes mellitus (scleredema diabeticorum) (242).

HISTOLOGY (FIGURE 6-3A, B):
■ Normal epidermis (sometimes effacement of the rete ridges)
■ Thickened dermis with collagen extending to the subcutaneous tissue
■ Increased spaces between large collagen bundles (this space results from increased deposition of hyaluronic acid in the dermis, which is more noticeable in the deep dermis)

DIFFERENTIAL DIAGNOSIS:
■ The main differential diagnosis includes scleromyxedema; however, the presence of acellular fibrosis in dermis contrasts with the marked fibroblastic proliferation seen in scleromyxedema.
■ Also, due to the thickening of dermis morphea/scleroderma may be included in the differential diagnosis; however, the latter usually shows a characteristic deep patchy inflammatory response.

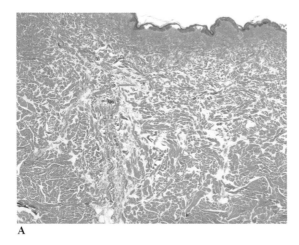
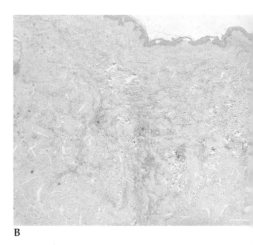

A   B

FIGURE 6-3 *Scleredema*
A. Thickened dermis with collagen extending to the subcutaneous tissue (note the spaces between large collagen bundles). **B.** Alcian blue (pH 2.5) shows increase amount of mucin in dermis.

Reticular erythematous mucinosis (REM) is a rare chronic dermatosis typically characterized by reticular macular erythema on the central area of the chest and back of young to middle-aged women. The pathogenesis and etiology of REM is unknown; however, some factors have been reportedly associated such as viral processes, immune diseases, and exposure to sunlight. There may be progression to cutaneous lupus erythematosus (240, 243).

HISTOLOGY: (FIGURE 6-4A, B)
- Epidermis is usually normal
- Mild superficial and mid-dermal perivascular lymphohistiocytic infiltrate (sometimes a perifollicular infiltrate)
- Sometimes a deep perivascular extension, restricted to the region of the eccrine glands
- Variable amounts of mucin deposition in upper and mid dermis (in chronic lesions it is sometimes absent)
- Fragmentation of elastic fibers
- The mucin material stains with colloidal iron and Alcian blue at pH 2.5

DIFFERENTIAL DIAGNOSIS:
- The main differential diagnosis of REM is with lupus erythematosus and PMLE.
- REM usually lacks the epidermal changes seen in LE; however, the tumid variant of LE can sometimes be impossible to distinguish based on histology alone, needing adjuvant studies such as serologic studies and DIF.
- In PMLE, the mucin deposition is not as striking and when seen is mainly located in the papillary dermis. Perifollicular inflammation is not seen in PMLE and epidermal changes (spongiosis and sometimes mild hydropic changes) and subepidermal edema are characteristic in PMLE. And to complicate things further, some authors consider that all these three entities are the same, i.e., tumid lupus.

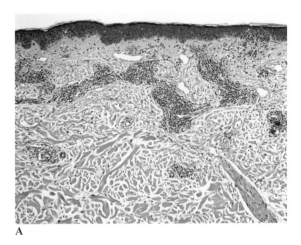
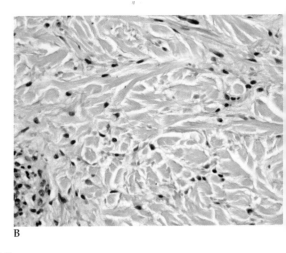

A   B

FIGURE 6-4 *Reticular Erythematous Mucinosis (REM)*
A. The biopsy shows a superficial perivascular and mid dermal moderately intense, lymphohistiocytic inflammation. Focal mucin deposition is noted in superficial dermis.
B. Higher magnification showing increased mucin deposition in interstitial dermis.

Digital mucous cysts are benign cysts of the digits, typically located on the hands at the distal interphalangeal joints, although they may also involve the toes. The etiology of these cysts is uncertain but may be secondary to mucoid degeneration after trauma (244).

HISTOLOGY (FIGURE 6-5):
- ◼ It shows a pseudocyst with a fibrous capsule with often a partial mesothelial lining, but not a true cyst wall.
- ◼ It often shows a myxomatous stroma with scattered fibroblasts.
- ◼ The overlying surface epithelium demonstrates compact hyperkeratosis with a collarette of hyperplastic epidermis.

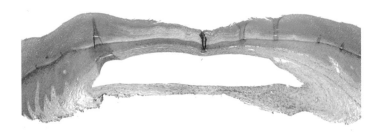

FIGURE 6-5 *Digital Mucous Cyst*
Pseudocyst lined by a fibrous capsule.

Mucocele results from the rupture of a duct of a minor salivary gland with extravasation of mucus into the submucosal tissues, most commonly on the lower lip. They may also develop in the buccal mucosa or tongue. Mucoceles are found mostly in young adults.

HISTOLOGY (FIGURE 6-6):
- **Two Histologic Variants:**
  A. Cystic structure with a surrounding, poorly defined lining of macrophages, fibroblasts, and capillaries. There is no epithelium lining the cyst.
  B. Granulation and fibrous tissue containing mucin-filled spaces with macrophages engulfing mucin.
- Numerous neutrophils and some eosinophils are present in the cystic spaces or in the stroma of both types.

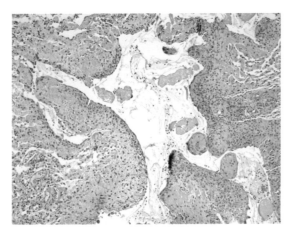

FIGURE 6-6 *Mucocele*
Cystic lesion lined by fibroblasts and macrophages. Note the mucin within the cystic cavity.

FOCAL DERMAL MUCINOSIS

It is an asymptomatic flesh colored papule or nodule occurring commonly on face, trunk or extremities of adults. It is thought that the increased amounts of mucin are produced by fibroblasts (245).

HISTOLOGY (FIGURE 6-7A, B):

- Dome-shaped dermal nodule with variable replacement of collagen bundles by mucin (the mucin may be localized to the upper dermis or extend through the full thickness of the dermis).
- Spindle-shaped fibroblasts within the mucinous areas (increase in small blood vessels).
- The histologic appearance may mimic the early stages of a digital mucous cyst.
- The mucin stains with colloidal iron and Alcian blue at pH 2.5.

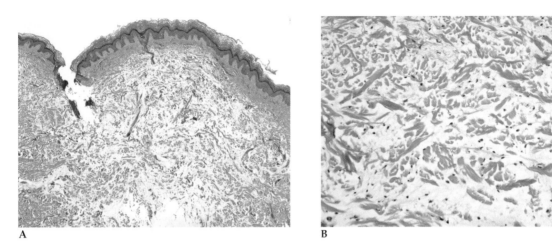

FIGURE 6-7 *Focal Dermal Mucinosis*
A. Dome-shaped dermal nodule with mucin deposition in reticular dermis. **B.** Higher magnification shows mucin deposition with scattered fibroblasts.

AMYLOIDOSIS

Amyloid may be deposited in virtually any organ, under many different clinical settings. Amyloid deposition may be systemic or may be localized like in rubbed skin from degeneration of keratinocytes without systemic involvement (246, 247).

Primary Systemic Amyloidosis: Cutaneous involvement is common in this type of amyloidosis and it is closely associated with immunocytic dyscrasias, particularly multiple myeloma. The fibrillar amyloid protein is composed of immunoglobulin light chains (AL type). It is most commonly seen in older patients and clinically presents with waxy purpuric macules and papules (hemorrhage) involving the hands and the periorbital skin. Skin lesions occur early in the disease course and their presence may be an important clue to an underlying B cell neoplasm.

Secondary Systemic Amyloidosis (AA Type): It is associated with a number of chronic inflammatory diseases such as tuberculosis, leprosy, mycosis fungoides, rheumatoid arthritis, familial Mediterranean fever, etc. Skin lesions are rare in secondary systemic amyloidosis. The fibrillar component is amyloid A protein (AA). Secondary amyloidosis may occur following hemodialysis, in which the protein fibril deposited is β2-microglobulin.

Nodular Amyloidosis: It is a rare form of localized amyloidosis that presents as nodules, often on the extremities or face and is most commonly seen in females. In at least 15% of cases, the patient will subsequently develop systemic amyloidosis; thus, patients with nodular deposits of amyloid should be carefully evaluated for systemic disease or progression to a lymphoproliferative disorders. The fibrillar component may be composed of AA, AL, or IAPP (islet amyloid polypeptide) amyloid (248).

Lichen and Macular Amyloidosis: These two dermatoses are considered as different manifestations of the same process. In contrast to systemic amyloidosis, they are localized to the skin and do not involve other organs. The fibrillar component is derived from keratinocytes and designated as AK (amyloid keratin). Lichen amyloidosis is characterized by discrete, pruritic, reddish brown papules that are most commonly seen on the shins. Macular amyloidosis is characterized by pruritic gray-brown macular lesions (rippled appearance) that are most commonly seen on the upper back (249, 250).

HISTOLOGY:

■ **Systemic and Nodular Amyloidosis:** It reveals dermal deposits of eosinophilic, amorphous hyaline material. The deposits form nodules or masses and also have a predilection for blood vessel walls and adnexal structures. Within the subcutaneous tissue, amyloid tends to be deposited around fat cells (**Figure 6-8A**).

■ **Macular Amyloidosis and Lichen Amyloidosis:** The deposits are subtle, and characterized by small, amorphous eosinophilic deposits within the superficial papillary dermis. Subepidermal clefting above the deposits rarely occurs. Pigmented cells are often seen within the dermal deposits and its presence is an important clue to the diagnosis of primary cutaneous amyloidosis. Lichen amyloidosis histologic manifestations of chronic rubbing are seen, namely, acanthosis, hypergranulosis, and hyperkeratosis (mimicking lichen simplex chronicus) (**Figure 6-8B–D**).

■ Since the source of amyloid in lichen and macular amyloidosis is keratin from damaged keratinocytes, these deposits are positive with immunohistochemical studies with anti-keratin antibodies (LP34 clone which detects CK5, 6, and 18).

■ Amyloid will display apple-green birefringence after Congo red staining, and it is also positive with crystal violet and thioflavine T stains.

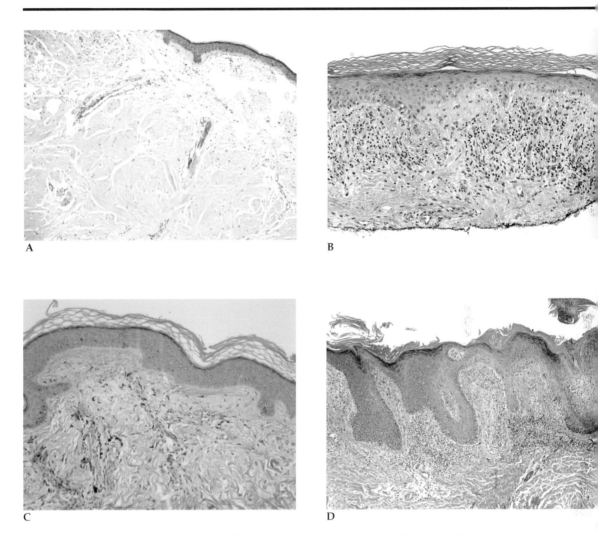

FIGURE 6-8 A. *Systemic amyloidosis.* Dermal deposits of eosinophilic amorphous hyaline material forming nodules. Also, there is deposition around blood vessel walls and adnexal structures. **B.** *Macular amyloidosis.* Note the small amorphous eosinophilic deposits within the superficial papillary dermis admixed with rare melanophages. **C.** *Macular amyloidosis.* Higher magnification showing the amorphous eosinophilic deposits with pigmented melanophages. **D.** *Lichen amyloidosis.* Acanthosis, hypergranulosis, and hyperkeratosis along with small amorphous eosinophilic deposits within the papillary dermis.

COLLOID MILIUM

Colloid milium clinically presents as multiple, translucent papules and plaques on sun-damaged skin, most commonly affecting the face and dorsum of the hands. There are four variants described: 1) *Adult-onset:* more common in middle-aged males and presents with numerous yellow dome-shaped papules. The head and neck area and dorsum of the hands are sites of predilection. Often there is a history of exposure to excessive sunlight and/or petroleum-based products, 2) *Colloid degeneration (paracolloid):* it presents as nodular and/or plaque-like areas, usually in chronically sun-exposed skin, particularly the face, 3) *Juvenile form:* it is very rare and clinically presents with papules or plaques usually on the face and neck, prior to puberty, 4) *Pigmented form:* this is found as dark clustered and/or confluent papules on the face, following the use of hydroquinone bleaching creams (251, 252).

HISTOLOGY (FIGURE 6-9):

- **Adult-Onset:** It shows nodular masses of homogeneous eosinophilic material in the upper and mid dermis (it may expand the papillary dermis), usually sparing the upper papillary dermis (grenz zone). Fissures and clefts are seen and fibroblasts may be aligned along the edges of these fissures. Solar elastosis is marked and adnexal structures are well preserved.
- **Colloid Degeneration (Paracolloid):** It shows amorphous dermal collagen with small fissures and clefts extending into dermis.
- **Juvenile Form:** In most areas there is no grenz zone and the islands of amorphous colloid are opposed to the basal layer of the epidermis. Solar elastosis is usually absent.
- **Pigmented Form:** Similar to other types of colloid milium but there is usually a light-golden pigmentation similar to ochronosis.
- Colloid milium is difficult to differentiate from amyloid under light microscopy alone. Both are positive for PAS stain; however, colloid is usually negative for the crystal violet stain (it may be focally positive). Colloid milium may also show focal green birefringence with Congo red stain.

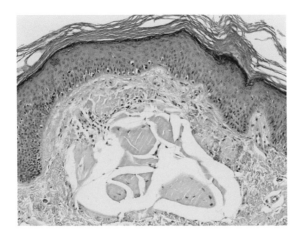

FIGURE 6-9 *Colloid Milium* A nodular mass of homogeneous eosinophilic material in the upper dermis with a grenz zone (note the fissures and clefts).

Lipoid proteinosis is a rare autosomal recessive dermatosis that is characterized by the deposition of an amorphous hyaline material in the skin and viscera. It presents in infancy with hoarseness ("hoarse cry") due to laryngeal infiltration; there are also recurrent skin infections. Waxy papules and plaques develop progressively over several years on the face, scalp, neck, and extremities. The disease typically follows a slowly progressive course and any organ may be involved. Lipoid proteinosis results from mutations in the gene encoding extracellular matrix protein 1 (ECM1) on chromosome 1q21 (253, 254).

HISTOLOGY:
- The early phase shows an eosinophilic hyaline thickening of papillary dermal capillaries.
- In advanced lesions there is epidermal hyperkeratosis and the papillary dermis is widened by hyaline material arranged perpendicular to the basement membrane zone. Also, hyaline deposits may be arranged around the adnexal structures and arrector pili muscles. The deposits around blood vessels may have an "onion-skin" appearance.
- The hyaline material stains positively with PAS (diastase resistant) and colloidal iron, Alcian blue (pH 2.5).

DIFFERENTIAL DIAGNOSIS:
- The differential diagnosis of lipoid proteinosis is mainly with erythropoietic protoporphyria (EP); however, the deposits in the EP are more limited (around the vessels and not around adnexal structures).

XANTHOMATOSIS

Xanthomas are defined as the accumulation of lipid-laden macrophages. Their recognition is important because they may be associated with underlying defects in lipid metabolism or other disorders. Xanthomas can be further subdivided on the basis of their clinical morphology, anatomical distribution, and mode of development.

Xanthelasmas: They are the most common of the xanthomas and occur most frequently around the eyes, characterized by whitish yellow plaques that are frequently bilateral. In approximately 50% of cases patients have underlying hypercholesterolemia.

Plane Xanthomas: Involvement of the palmar creases is characteristic of type III dysbetalipoproteinemia. They can also be associated with secondary hyperlipidemias. Generalized (diffuse) plane xanthomas usually involve the trunk and neck and the majority of patients are normolipidemic; however, they may be associated with monoclonal gammopathy and hyperlipidemia, particularly hypertriglyceridemia (255).

Tuberous Xanthomas: Painless, red-yellow nodules typically involving pressure points such as elbows, knees, buttocks, and posterior thighs. The lesions can coalesce to form multilobated tumors. Tuberous xanthomas are particularly associated with familial hyperlipoproteinemia (type III).

Eruptive Xanthomas: Rapid onset of numerous reddish-yellow papules, especially in buttocks or thighs. They are associated with elevated plasma chylomicrons (diabetes mellitus), alcohol, or the use of exogenous estrogens. Other associations include hypertriglyceridemia, particularly that associated with types I, IV, and V (256).

Tendinous Xanthomas: Hard, skin-colored nodules which develop slowly over time, and usually on the extensor tendons of the hands, feet, and the Achilles tendon. Sometimes they are associated with trauma. They are most commonly associated with heterozygous familial hypercholesterolemia.

Verruciform Xanthomas: They predominantly occur in the oral cavity of adults, although lesions have also been reported on the genital area. They usually present in normolipemic patients as a single warty papillomatous yellow lesion (257).

HISTOLOGY (FIGURE 6-10A–C):
- All xanthomas are characterized by foamy cells which are macrophages that have engulfed lipid droplets.
- Cholesterol clefts and stromal fibrosis are frequently noted in tuberous and tendinous xanthomas.
- Touton giant cells are sometimes present.
- Eruptive xanthomas are most likely to have extracellular deposition of triglycerides and more lymphocytes and neutrophils.
- Verruciform xanthomas show a verruca-like architecture with often exocytosis of neutrophils into the upper layers of the epithelium. The papillary dermis is filled with numerous large xanthoma cells admixed with variable numbers of lymphocytes, plasma cells, neutrophils, and eosinophils beneath and between the xanthoma cells.

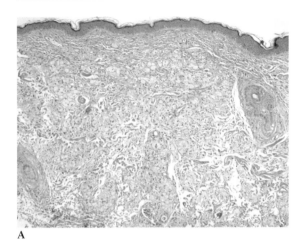

A

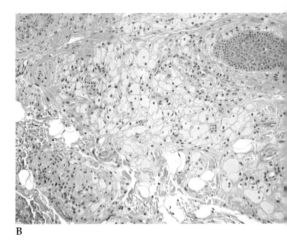

B

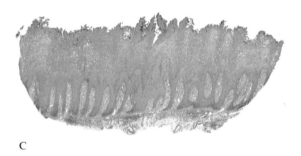

C

FIGURE 6-10 *Xanthoma*
A. The biopsy shows a nodular proliferation of foamy histiocytes filling dermis.
B. Many foamy macrophages in dermis. **C.** Verruciform xanthomas. Verruca-like architecture and papillary dermis is filled with numerous large xanthoma cells.

GOUT

Gout is a disorder of uric acid metabolism that leads to the deposition of monosodium urate crystals. Uric acid crystal deposits, sometimes referred to as gouty tophi, are typically located in small joints, particularly the great toe. The ear, although less commonly involved, is also a characteristic site. Uric acid crystals are dissolved during routine formalin fixation and processing for H&E-stained sections (258).

HISTOLOGY (FIGURE 6-11A, B):

■ Pale white, radially arranged amorphous material with a feathery or fibrillar border surrounded by a granulomatous reaction.
■ Slender, slit like clear spaces represent the outline of the dissolved crystals.
■ Calcification may be a late complication.
■ Alcohol fixation and anhydrous processing preserve the crystal structure. Polarization microscopy demonstrates needle-shaped brown crystals that are doubly refractile.

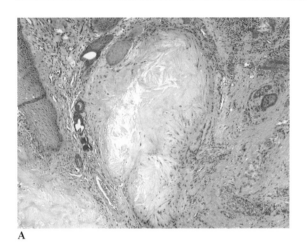
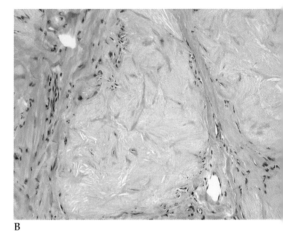

A

B

FIGURE 6-11 *Gout*
A. Grayish amorphous material with a fibrillar border surrounded by macrophages
(note the slit like clear spaces that represent the outline of the dissolved crystals).
B. Higher magnification showing the fibrillary appearance of these deposits.

CALCINOSIS CUTIS

Calcinosis cutis is a term used to describe a group of disorders in which calcium deposits form in the skin. The underlying cause may not be discernible on light microscopic evaluation; therefore, careful clinical evaluation, such as for causes of hypercalcemia, should be instituted when appropriate. Several clinical variations have been identified (251).

Dystrophic Calcification: It refers to calcification of previously damaged tissue, and by definition, patients have normal serum calcium or phosphate level and internal organs are spared. Dystrophic calcification may occur in the setting of trauma, infections, tumors, connective tissue diseases, particularly dermatomyositis, scleroderma (especially CREST syndrome), and lupus erythematosus.

Metastatic Calcinosis: Arises in the setting of abnormal calcium or phosphate metabolism. Most commonly, patients have hypercalcemia due to hyperparathyroidism, paraneoplastic hypercalcemia, hyperphosphatemia, hypervitaminosis D, milk-alkali syndrome, renal failure, etc.

Tumoral Calcinosis: It is characterized by the presence of large multiple deposits of calcium hydroxyapatite that most commonly involve the periarticular soft tissue on the extensor aspect of large joints. This is more commonly seen in African Americans.

Familial Tumoral Calcinosis: It is an autosomal recessive disorder caused by hyperphosphatemia secondary to the increased renal reabsorption of phosphate. Some patients have mutations in the GALNT3 gene on chromosome 2q24–q31.

Idiopathic Scrotal Calcinosis Cutis: Single or multiple lesions develop in the scrotal skin in children or young adults. Calcification may occur after trauma and some cases may be secondary to ruptured follicular cysts.

Subepidermal Calcified Nodule: These lesions usually develop in early childhood and are typically solitary, though multiple lesions can also be present. The nodules most commonly occur on the face, though they may occur anywhere.

Iatrogenic Calcinosis Cutis: Calcification generally is located at the site of an invasive procedure, as in intravenous administration of solutions containing calcium or phosphate and in tumor lysis syndrome.

HISTOLOGY (FIGURE 6-12):
- In H&E-stained sections, calcium stains deep blue to purple. Calcium is refractile and frequently demonstrates a "cracked" or fragmented appearance.
- Calcification is occasionally present as fine pale blue and gray granular material.
- When necessary, the Von Kossa or alizarin red stain may be used to confirm the presence of calcification.
- In tumoral calcinosis the subcutaneous deposits tend to be large and dense.
- In subepidermal calcified nodule there is often overlying pseudoepitheliomatous hyperplasia, associated with transepidermal elimination of some calcified granules (transepidermal elimination of calcium deposits is uncommon in the other forms).

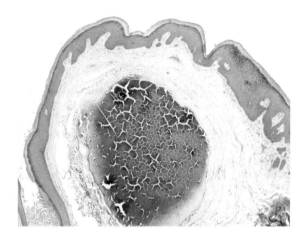

FIGURE 6-12 *Calcinosis Cutis*
Intradermal calcification. This example represents a case of scrotal calcinosis.

OCHRONOSIS

Two types of ochronosisis have been described, endogenous and exogenous. Ochronosis refers to the bluish black discoloration of certain tissues, such as the ear cartilage and the ocular tissue. Endogenous ochronosis is a rare autosomal recessive metabolic disorder caused by deficiency of homogentisic acid oxidase, the only enzyme capable of catabolizing homogentisic acid. The disease results in the accumulation and deposition of homogentisic acid in the cartilage, eyelids, forehead, cheeks, axilla, genital region, buccal mucosa, tendons, etc. In exogenous ochronosis, there is bluish black pigmentation of cartilage after iatrogenic use of agents, such as hydroquinone, phenol, trinitrophenol and benzene (251, 259).

HISTOLOGY (FIGURE 6-13):

- Yellowish brown pigmented bodies alkaptonuria in the dermis that are sharply defined in a crescentic, vermiform, or in banana shape.
- Fragmented fibers and small pigmented deposits (sometimes within macrophages).
- Colloid milium-like foci can often be seen in the hydroquinone-induced lesions.
- Transfollicular elimination of ochronotic fibers.

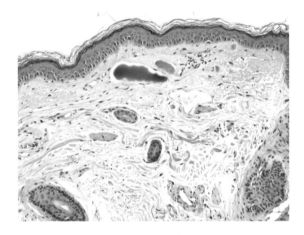

FIGURE 6-13 *Exogenous Ochronosis*
Brown pigmented bodies in the dermis that are banana shaped.

ARGYRIA (SILVER DEPOSITION)

Argyria is the systemic accumulation of silver, resulting from prolonged contact with or ingestion of silver salts. Clinically, it is characterized by a gray-black staining of the skin (most marked in sun-exposed areas) and mucous membranes after silver deposition in the dermis. Silver may be deposited in the skin either from industrial exposure or as a result of medications containing silver salts (260).

HISTOLOGY:
- Small, round, brown-black granules appear singly or in clusters mainly around the basement membrane zone of sweat glands.
- The granules are also found in elastic fibers (papillary dermis) and to a lesser degree in the connective tissue sheaths around the pilosebaceous follicles and around the pili erector muscle.
- They are best visualized as strikingly refractile with dark-field illumination ("stars in heaven pattern").

Selected Genodermatosis

7

INCONTINENTIA PIGMENTI

Incontinentia pigmenti (IP) is a rare X-linked dominant genodermatosis with cutaneous, neurologic, ophthalmologic, and dental manifestations. IP is almost always lethal in males and thus more than 95% of reported cases of IP occur in females. It is associated with mutations in the IKK-gamma gene, also known as NEMO, which maps to Xq28. Cutaneous symptoms are present at birth or occur within the first weeks of life. The cutaneous manifestations usually appear in a characteristic chronologic sequence (vesicular, verrucous, and hyperpigmented stages). Other systemic clinical manifestations, including ocular defects, CNS abnormalities, and dental abnormalities, may not be apparent until infancy or childhood (261, 262).

HISTOLOGY (FIGURE 7-1):
■ **First Stage (Vesicular):** Eosinophilic spongiosis and scattered dyskeratotic cells. Also, intraepidermal vesicles filled with eosinophils.
■ **Second Stage (Verrucous):** Epidermal hyperkeratosis, acanthosis and a subtle irregular papillomatosis with many dyskeratotic cells. Mild vacuolar damage along with rare eosinophils.
■ **Third Stage (Hyperpigmented):** Characteristic pigment incontinence within papillary dermis. Mild vacuolar changes with rare dyskeratotic cells.

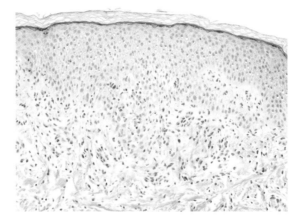

FIGURE 7-1 *Incontinentia Pigmenti "First Stage"* Eosinophilic spongiosis with rare dyskeratotic cells.

Porokeratosis is a clonal disorder of keratinization characterized by one or more atrophic patches surrounded by a peripheral distinctive threadlike ring. Porokeratosis was originally known as a familial disease with autosomal dominant inheritance; however, numerous non-familial cases have now been reported. Several risk factors have been described in the development of porokeratosis including genetic inheritance, ultraviolet radiation, and immunosuppression. There are five clinical variants of porokeratosis: classic porokeratosis of Mibelli, disseminated superficial actinic porokeratosis (DSAP), porokeratosis palmaris et plantaris disseminata, linear porokeratosis, and punctate porokeratosis. Porokeratoma is a recently described solitary plaque or nodule, with sometimes a verrucous appearance, with a predilection for the distal extremities of middle-aged to elderly males (263, 264).

HISTOLOGY (FIGURE 7-2):

- In all types of porokeratosis the hallmark is the presence of a cornoid lamella (layered column of parakeratosis within the stratum corneum).
- Most of the time the cornoid lamellae is obliquely oriented and underneath there is focal absence of granular layer.
- Dyskeratotic cells may be seen subjacent in the upper levels of epidermis.
- In porokeratosis of Mibelli there is invagination of the epidermis at the site of the cornoid lamella.
- DSAP may show a lichenoid inflammatory response with focal interface changes. Adjacent epidermis shows actinic changes.

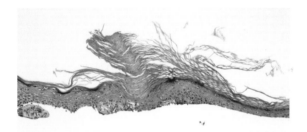

FIGURE 7-2 *Porokeratosis*
Layered column of parakeratosis within the stratum corneum (cornoid lamella).

ICHTHYOSIS

Ichthyosis refers to a rare group of skin disorders characterized by the presence of excessive amounts of dry surface scales. It is regarded as a disorder of keratinization due to abnormal epidermal metabolism. There are different types of ichthyosis including: ichthyosis vulgaris, X-linked ichthyosis, lamellar ichthyosis, congenital ichthyosiform erythroderma (CIE), epidermolytic hyperkeratosis (bullous ichthyosiform erythroderma), acquired ichthyosis, etc.

Ichthyosis Vulgaris: It is the most common form; an autosomal dominant disorder that usually starts in early childhood. White scales are present on trunk, abdomen, buttocks, and legs. This disorder is commonly associated with atopic dermatitis and keratosis pilaris. The flexural areas are spared. The molecular marker affected is profilaggrin, a high molecular weight filaggrin precursor, the major protein of keratohyalin granules (265, 266).

X-linked Ichthyosis: It is the second most common type, inherited as X-linked recessive trait. This disorder is present at birth or develops in the first few months of life as generalized scaling that is most prominent over the extremities, neck, trunk, and buttocks. The flexural creases, palms, and soles are spared. There may be corneal opacities and mental changes. This disorder is characterized by a deficiency of steroid sulfatase (STS), a gene located on the distal short arm of the X chromosome (Xp22.3) (267, 268).

Lamellar Ichthyosis: It is a rare, autosomal recessive heterogeneous disorder caused by mutations involving multiple genetic loci. The newborn is encased in a collodion membrane that sheds within 2 weeks. The shedding of the membrane reveals generalized scaling with fine or plate-like pattern, resembling fish skin (hence the name icthyosis). The scaling of the skin involves the whole body with no sparing of the flexural creases. Type 1 maps to band 14q11.2 and is caused by mutations in the gene for keratinocyte transglutaminase 1. Type 2, which is clinically indistinguishable from type 1, maps to band 2q33-q35 (269).

Congenital Ichthyosiform Erythroderma (CIE): This disorder is a milder, autosomal recessive form of ichthyosis. Neonates with CIE are referred to as collodion babies. Children and adults show generalized thin white scales. Other manifestations commonly seen in this disorder include persistent ectropion and scarring alopecia. CIE is caused by mutations in the genes coding for transglutaminase 1, 12R-lipoxygenase, and/or lipoxygenase 3.

Epidermolytic Hyperkeratosis (Bullous Ichthyosiform Erythroderma): This is a rare, autosomal dominant disorder, usually severe and characterized at birth by widespread erythroderma, severe scaling and some blistering. The cause is a mutation in the keratin genes (i.e., KRT1, KRT10) (270).

Acquired Ichthyosis: It is seen in adults and clinically presents as small, white, fishlike scales more commonly seen on the extremities but may be generalized. This form of ichthyosis may be associated with systemic illness (lupus, diabetes, sarcoidosis, HIV infection, hypothyroidism, chronic hepatitis, malnutrition), malignancies (Hodgkin lymphoma, leukemia), bone marrow transplantation, drug reactions, etc. (265).

HISTOLOGY:

- **Ichthyosis Vulgaris:** The stratum corneum shows compact orthokeratosis with mild to moderate hyperkeratosis and associated with a markedly reduced or absent granular layer. The epidermis shows normal thickness and there is follicular dilatation with hyperkeratosis. Sebaceous glands are atrophic (**Figure 7-3**).
- **X-linked Ichthyosis:** Epidermal acanthosis with marked orthokeratosis and hyperkeratosis (possible foci of parakeratosis). The granular layer is usually thickened but can be thinned.
- **Lamellar Ichthyosis:** Mild to moderate hyperkeratosis with normal or thickened granular layer. Epidermal acanthosis and papillomatosis.
- **Congenital Ichthyosiform Erythroderma (CIE):** Similar to lamellar ichthyosis but with more discernible parakeratosis.
- **Epidermolytic Hyperkeratosis (Bullous Ichthyosiform Erythroderma):** Massive hyperkeratosis with a thickened granular layer and coarse keratohyaline granules. The epidermis shows characteristic acanthosis with epidermolysis.
- **Acquired Ichthyosis:** The histologic changes are similar to ichthyosis vulgaris, such as compact orthokeratosis with hyperkeratosis and a reduced or absent granular layer.

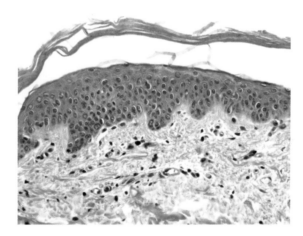

FIGURE 7-3 *Ichthyosis Vulgaris*
Orthokeratosis with hyperkeratosis associated with a markedly reduced granular layer.

CONFLUENT AND RETICULATED PAPILLOMATOSIS

Confluent and reticulated papillomatosis (CARP) is a rare dermatosis that is characterized by hyperkeratotic papules, usually located on the trunk, and more commonly seen in young patients. The lesions coalesce to form confluent plaques centrally and a reticular pattern peripherally. CARP has been thought to represent a genodermatosis, an endocrine disturbance, a variant of acanthosis nigricans, a disorder of keratinization, or a reaction to fungi (Pityrosporum orbiculare) (271, 272).

HISTOLOGY (FIGURE 7-4):
- The epidermis shows undulations with compact hyperkeratosis and papillomatosis.
- Papillomatosis may be absent.
- Decreased or absent granular cell layer.
- The stratum spinosum varies from acanthotic to atrophic.
- Mild hyperpigmentation of basal keratinocytes.
- Pityrosporum yeasts in the stratum corneum.

DIFFERENTIAL DIAGNOSIS:
- Acanthosis nigricans may show similar features; however, in CARP the changes are not as developed. Also, the presence of fungus, if encountered, will favor CARP.

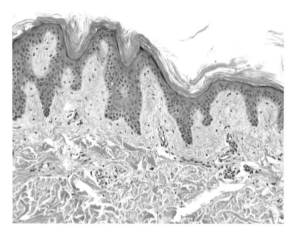

FIGURE 7-4 *Confluent and Reticulated Papillomatosis (CARP)*
Epidermal papillomatosis with mild pigmentation of the basal layer.

This is a rare genodermatosis that clinically is characterized by multiple, localized, symmetrical, flat-topped papules on the dorsum of the hands and fingers and less commonly on the feet, forearms, and legs. This disorder has an autosomal dominant mode of inheritance. Lesions identical to those of acrokeratosis verruciformis are also observed in many patients with acral Darier disease. ATP2A2 encoding the SERCA2 pump has been identified as the defective gene in Darier disease and rarely in acrokeratosis verruciformis (273, 274).

HISTOLOGY (FIGURE 7-5):

■ Hyper(ortho)keratosis, regular acanthosis and papillomatosis with a prominent granular layer ("church spire" architecture)

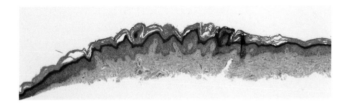

FIGURE 7-5 *Acrokeratosis Verruciformis of Hopf*
The biopsy shows hyperkeratosis, acanthosis, and papillomatosis with a prominent granular layer, typically having a "church spire" appearance.

Alopecias

8

Alopecia Areata

Alopecia areata (AA) is a not uncommon dermatosis that most commonly affects patients between the ages of 15 and 40. "Clinically, it presents with sudden onset as one of more, asymptomatic, localized, non-scarring hairless patches, usually on the scalp; however, it can affect any hair-bearing area." AA may spontaneously regress or may progress to involve the entire scalp (alopecia totalis) and more rarely all body hair (alopecia universalis). AA can be associated with diseases such as atopic dermatitis, diabetes, Hashimoto thyroiditis, Addison disease, idiopathic primary hypophysitis, vitiligo, SLE, etc. (275, 276).

HISTOLOGY (FIGURE 8-1):

- The anagen follicles show a peribulbar infiltrate of lymphocytes (swarm of bees pattern) admixed with rare eosinophils, plasma cells, and pigment incontinence. However, this pattern is not always observed, especially in the chronic phase of the disease.
- The peribulbar inflammatory response tends to decrease as the affected hair progresses to the telogen phase.
- A significant decrease in terminal hairs is associated with an increase in vellus hairs.
- A fibrous tract extends along the site of the previous follicle into the subcutis.

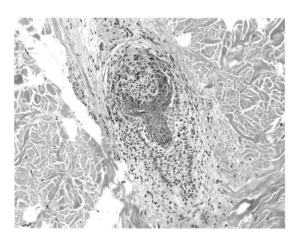

FIGURE 8-1 *Alopecia Areata*
Peribulbar infiltrate of lymphocytes in a "swarm-of-bees" pattern.

Androgenetic Alopecia

Androgenetic alopecia (common baldness) is a very common disorder that is genetically determined and progresses through the gradual conversion of terminal hairs into vellus hairs (reduced terminal-to-vellus hair ratio). It affects roughly 50% of men and also a number of older women. Clinically, it presents as a progressive replacement of terminal hairs by fine vellus hairs with hair loss in characteristic geographical areas of the scalp (277, 278).

HISTOLOGY:
- There is progressive miniaturization of hair follicles and their shafts toward vellus formation.
- There is also an increase in the number of telogen and catagen hairs relative to the number of anagen hairs (mild increase in telogen-to-anagen ratio).

Trichotillomania

Trichotillomania is a traumatic alopecia that results from repetitive hair manipulations. It is more commonly seen in women and clinically shows a geometrical shape and incomplete non-scarring alopecia more commonly seen in the crown and occipital scalp (279).

HISTOLOGY (FIGURE 8-2A, B):
- Increased numbers of catagen hairs associated usually with the presence of early and late anagen hairs
- Presence of empty follicles (pulled hair shafts)
- Trichomalacia (deformed hair shafts)
- Pigmented casts

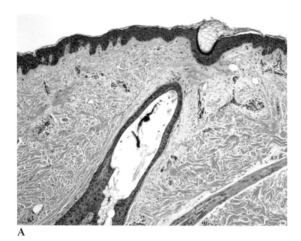 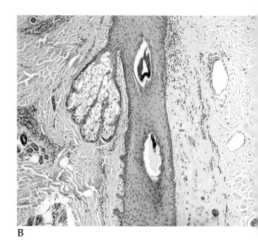

A B

FIGURE 8-2 *Trichotillomania*
A. The biopsy shows an empty follicle with distorted hair and pigmented casts.
B. Higher magnification of the pigmented casts.

Telogen Effluvium

Telogen effluvium is a common reactive dermatosis caused by a metabolic or hormonal stress or by medications that are clinically characterized by diffuse thinning and shedding of the scalp hair, often with an acute onset. It usually presents 3 months after the stressful event.

HISTOLOGY:
- Increased number of telogen hair follicles and follicular stellae (usually seen in deep dermis and subcutaneous fat)
- The total number of hair follicles is normal.

Lichen Planopilaris

Lichen planopilaris (LPP) is a rare cause of scarring alopecia. It is most commonly seen in adult women and the scalp is often the only site involved; however, can be generalized in about half of the cases. LPP can be multifocal or diffuse, often starting on the central scalp (43, 280).

HISTOLOGY (FIGURE 8-3):
- Lichenoid inflammatory response involving the basal layer of the follicular epithelium (usually associated with perifollicular lymphohistiocytic infiltrate).
- Dyskeratotic keratinocytes are seen in the follicular epithelium with minimal involvement of the interfollicular epidermis (however, it can be involved in up to one-third of cases with scalp involvement).
- The late stage shows sclerotic perifollicular fibrosis and loss of hair follicles that are replaced by linear tracts of fibrosis.

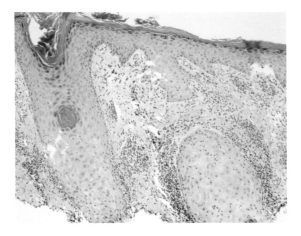

FIGURE 8-3 *Lichen Planopilaris*
Lichenoid inflammatory response involving the basal layer of the follicular epithelium. Note the perifollicular fibrosis.

Pseudopelade of Brocq

Pseudopelade of Brocq is not a specific disease, but rather represents a pattern of scarring alopecia. Some authors believed that pseudopelade of Brocq was a unique entity; however, most authorities now believe that this disease represents the end stage of different forms of scarring alopecia. Clinically, it is more commonly seen in females over the age of 40 years and results in patches of hair loss (single or multiple) that have been described as resembling "footprints in the snow." This same exact pattern of alopecia can be found in end-stage DLE, LLP, and other forms of cicatricial alopecia.

HISTOLOGY:
- Mild lymphocytic infiltrate at the follicular infundibulum
- Reduced or absent sebaceous glands
- Perifollicular fibrosis (onion-skin pattern)
- In late stage, extensive fibrosis containing elastic tissue replace the hair follicles and sebaceous glands

Folliculitis Keloidalis Nuchae
(Acne Keloidalis Nuchae)

Folliculitis keloidalis nuchae is a rare idiopathic variant of scarring alopecia of the nape of the neck, restricted almost exclusively to adult African American males. Clinically, it presents with multiple follicular papules and pustules which enlarge, forming confluent, thickened plaques that eventually progress to hair loss (281, 282).

HISTOLOGY (FIGURE 8-4):
- Dense dermal hyalinized fibrosis with keloid formation is admixed with a chronic inflammatory cell infiltrate composed of numerous plasma cells (mainly around the follicular structures).
- Hair shafts in dermis are surrounded by microabscesses and/or foreign body giant cells.
- Sinus tracts may lead to the epidermal surface.

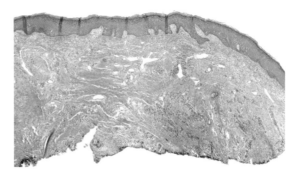

FIGURE 8-4 *Folliculitis Kelodalis Nuchae*
Dense dermal hyalinized fibrosis admixed with a chronic inflammatory composed of many plasma cells and loss of hair follicles.

Folliculitis Decalvans

Folliculitis decalvans is a form of scarring alopecia that clinically presents with recurrent crops of follicular pustules that lead to destruction of the follicle and consequent permanent hair loss. The exact cause of this condition is unknown, but in most cases Staphylococci is cultured from pustules (283).

HISTOLOGY (FIGURE 8-5A, B):
- The initial phase shows folliculitis and eventually destruction of the hair follicle ensues.
- The dermis surrounding the destroyed hair follicle shows a mixed inflammatory cell infiltrate and plasma cells can be increased in number.
- Scar tissue reaction in dermis

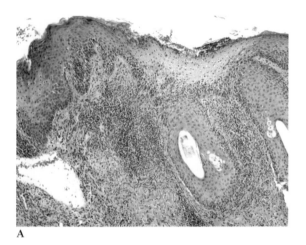 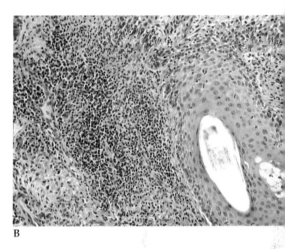

A   B

FIGURE 8-5 *Folliculitis Decalvans*
A. The biopsy shows an intense inflammatory folliculitis in which the entire length of the follicle is surrounded by a dense inflammatory infiltrate. The infiltrate is mostly lymphohistiocytic but admixed with many plasma cells. **B.** Higher magnification shows many plasma cells admixed with the lymphohistiocytic infiltrate.

Alopecia Mucinosa (Follicular Mucinosis)

Alopecia mucinosa is a rare form of scarring alopecia that clinically presents as pruritic follicular papules and plaques. The scalp, face, and neck are the most commonly affected sites; however, lesions may appear anywhere. Three clinical variants of the disease have been described: 1) primary acute disorder of young patients that presents with one or several plaques or grouped follicular papules, usually limited to the face or scalp, 2) primary chronic disorder of older patients that presents with a wide distribution of follicular papules, plaques, and nodules on the face, trunk, and extremities, and 3) a secondary disorder associated with lymphoma or mycosis fungoides (15%–30% of cases) (284, 285).

HISTOLOGY (FIGURE 8-6):
- Follicular degeneration with the deposition of mucin within the hair follicles
- A perivascular, interstitial, and periadnexal lymphocytic inflammatory infiltrate admixed with histiocytes, plasma cells, and rare eosinophils
- In alopecia mucinosa secondary to lymphomas the lymphocytic infiltrate is heavier and nodular (with atypical lymphocytes) and sometimes has more plasma cells than in primary alopecia mucinosa

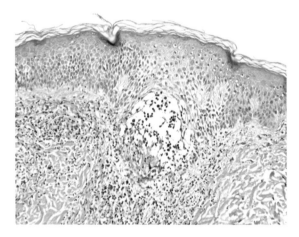

FIGURE 8-6 *Alopecia Mucinosa*
Degenerated hair follicle with mucin deposition and lymphocytic exocytosis.

Infectious Diseases of the Skin

9

BACTERIAL DISEASES
IMPETIGO
STAPHYLOCOCCAL SCALDED SKIN SYNDROME
ECTHYMA
CELLULITIS
CHANCROID
GRANULOMA INGUINALE
RHINOSCLEROMA
LEPROSY
SYPHILIS
LYME DISEASE (ERYTHEMA CHRONICUM MIGRANS)
BACILLARY ANGIOMATOSIS

FUNGAL DISEASES
DERMATOPHYTOSIS
TINEA VERSICOLOR
TINEA NIGRA
CHROMOMYCOSIS
PHAEOHYPHOMYCOSIS
SPOROTRICOSIS
CRYPTOCOCCOSIS
FUSARIOSIS
COCCIDIOMYCOSIS
BLASTOMYCOSIS
HISTOPLASMOSIS
PARACOCCIDIOIDOMYCOSIS
ZYGOMYCOSIS
ASPERGILLOSIS
RHINOSPORIDIOSIS
LOBOMYCOSIS

(continued)

(continued)

VIRAL AND CHLAMYDIAL DISEASES
HUMAN PAPILLOMAVIRUS INFECTION (WARTS)
HERPES INFECTIONS
MOLLUSCUM CONTAGIOSUM
ORF AND MILKER NODULE
GIANOTTI-CROSTI SYNDROME (PAPULAR ACRODERMATITIS OF CHILDHOOD)
LYMPHOGRANULOMA VENEREUM

PARASITIC AND ARTHROPOD-INDUCED DISEASES
LEISHMANIASIS
AMEBIASIS CUTIS
PROTOTHECOSIS
CYSTICERCOSIS
DIROFILARIASIS
ONCHOCERCASIS
CUTANEOUS LARVA MIGRANS
SCABIES
TUNGIASIS

Impetigo

Impetigo is a bacterial infection of the superficial layers of the epidermis. There are two types of impetigo: bullous impetigo and vesiculopustular "non-bullous" impetigo. Non-bullous impetigo is caused by Staphylococcus aureus and group A beta hemolytic streptococcus, and the bullous form is related exclusively to Staphylococcus aureus (phage group II) (286, 287).

HISTOLOGY (FIGURE 9-1):
- **Non-Bullous Impetigo:** Focal collection of subcorneal neutrophils
- **Bullous Impetigo:** Subcorneal bullae with scattered acantholytic cells and neutrophils
- Gram positive cocci

DIFFERENTIAL DIAGNOSIS:
- The differential diagnosis of bullous impetigo includes pustular psoriasis, subcorneal pustular dermatosis, AGEP, etc. Special stains are needed to detect the characteristic gram-positive cocci.

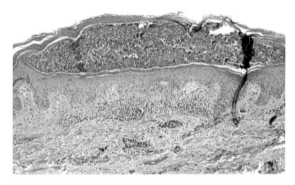

FIGURE 9-1 *Impetigo*
Subcorneal deposition of neutrophils.

Staphylococcal Scalded Skin Syndrome

Staphylococcal scalded skin syndrome (SSSS) is a toxin-mediated dermatitis that encompasses a spectrum of superficial blistering skin disorders. SSSS is caused by the release of two exotoxins (epidermolytic toxins A and B) from toxigenic strains of the bacteria Staphylococcus aureus. The disease predominantly affects healthy infants and children (<6 years) reflecting their inability to excrete the toxin. Also at risk are immuno-compromised patients and patients with renal failure. Clinically, SSSS begins with fever and a generalized red macular tender erythema followed by the development of large flaccid bullae involving particularly the head and neck, and trunk (288, 289).

HISTOLOGY (FIGURE 9-2):
- Splitting/clefting underneath the stratum corneum.
- Acantholytic cells and neutrophils may be seen within the clefting.
- In dermis, a mild lymphocytic infiltrate.

DIFFERENTIAL DIAGNOSIS:
- The main differential diagnosis includes pemphigus foliaceus (PF). In SSSS the dermal infiltrate is not as pronounced as in PF, and the DIF is negative.

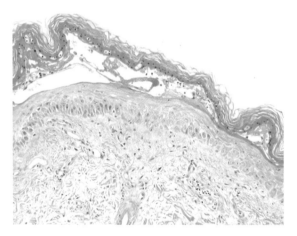

FIGURE 9-2 *Staphylococcal Scalded Skin Syndrome*
Splitting underneath the stratum corneum.

Ecthyma

Ecthyma is defined as presence of bacteria within the dermis. Ecthyma is usually caused by Group A streptococci *(Streptococcus pyogenes)*. Clinically, it arises on the lower extremities of children and presents as a shallow ulcer surrounded by erythema (sometimes can be multiple). *Ecthyma gangrenosum* is a variation of ecthyma usually seen in immunosuppressed individuals who develop a bacteremia with *Pseudomonas aeruginosa* and almost always represents a clinical sign of sepsis. It shows hemorrhagic pustules with surrounding erythema that evolve into necrotic ulcers (290).

HISTOLOGY:
- **Ecthyma:** Epidermal ulceration with a dense neutrophilic infiltrate in the reticular dermis. Gram stains should help in detecting the bacteria within the dermis.
- **Ecthyma Gangrenosum:** Necrosis of the epidermis and the upper dermis along with a mixed inflammatory infiltrate around the infarcted region. Necrotizing vasculitis with vascular thrombosis and lightly eosinophilic material corresponding to the clusters of *Pseudomonas* organisms. Gram-negative rods can be identified in the media and adventitia of the necrotic vessels and in interstitial dermis.

Cellulitis

Cellulitis is a non-necrotizing bacterial inflammation of the dermis that does not involve the fascia. Clinically, it is characterized by localized pain, swelling, tenderness, erythema, and warmth. The vast majority of cases are caused by *Streptococcus pyogenes* or *Staphylococcus aureus* (291).

HISTOLOGY:
- Most cases show only edema and a mild mixed neutrophilic/lymphocytic infiltrate. The bacteria may be sometimes identified with the special stains.

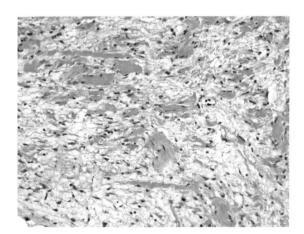

FIGURE 9-3 *Cellulitis*
The biopsy shows edema in reticular dermis along with a moderately dense, perivascular and interstitial infiltrate composed of lymphocytes, histiocytes, neutrophils, and rare eosinophils.

BACTERIAL DISEASES

Chancroid

Chancroid is a sexually transmitted disease caused by a gram-negative bacillus *Haemophilus ducreyi*. Clinically, it has a short incubation period and is characterized by the presence of painful irregular ulcers in the genital area and tender inguinal lymphadenopathy (292).

HISTOLOGY:
- Ulcerated epidermis
- Underneath the ulcer there are three distinct zones. The superficial zone shows neutrophils, fibrin, red blood cells, and necrosis. The second zone is wider and contains newly formed blood vessels with marked endothelial cell proliferation (the lumina of these vessels can be occluded). The deepest zone shows a dense infiltrate of plasma cells and lymphoid cells.
- Giemsa stain may show the organisms lying free and/or within histiocytes around the base of the ulcer.

Granuloma Inguinale

Granuloma inguinale (Donovanosis) is a sexually transmitted disease caused by a gram-negative bacillus, *Calymmatobacterium granulomatis*. The incubation period is from 2 to 4 weeks. Granuloma inguinale usually affects the skin and mucous membranes in the genital region, and presents as raised nodules that erode to form red velvety heaped-up ulcers, which gradually increase in size (293).

HISTOLOGY:
- The epidermis is ulcerated and shows acanthosis and pseudoepitheliomatous hyperplasia at the edges.
- A dense dermal infiltrate of histiocytes and plasma cells is present at the base of the ulcer.
- The macrophages are large and vacuolated and they contain intracellular bacilli (Donovan bodies) which are sometimes seen by Warthin–Starry or Giemsa stain.
- The best way to detect the organisms is by examining tissue smears with Wright or Giemsa stain.

Rhinoscleroma

Rhinoscleroma is a chronic granulomatous disorder of the nasal and oral mucosa. Rhinoscleroma is a result of infection by the gram-negative bacteria *Klebsiella rhinoscleromatis*. Rhinoscleroma is endemic to areas of Africa, Southeast Asia, Mexico, Central and South America, and Eastern Europe. Most often, the presentation is that of purulent sinusitis (294).

HISTOLOGY (FIGURE 9-4):
- Variable number of plasma cells with Russell bodies
- Large mononuclear histiocytes with vacuolated cytoplasm (Mikulicz cells)
- The organisms can be best seen in the cytoplasm of these cells by Warthin–Starry stain.

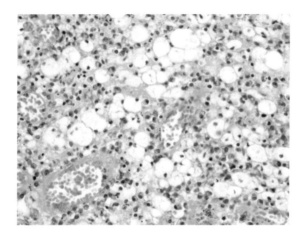

FIGURE 9-4 *Rhinoscleroma*
There are large mononuclear histiocytes with vacuolated cytoplasm (Mikulicz cells). Note the many plasma cells.

BACTERIAL DISEASES

Leprosy

Leprosy is a chronic granulomatous disease principally affecting the skin, nasal mucosa and peripheral nerves. Leprosy is caused by an acid fast bacteria *Mycobacterium leprae*. Leprosy is most prevalent in tropical countries and the principal mode of transmission is by spread of person to person through nasal secretions or droplets. Leprosy shows a wide spectrum of clinical presentations that correlate with the histopathological changes and the immune status of the patient. These include indeterminate, tuberculoid, lepromatous, borderline-tuberculoid, borderline, and borderline-lepromatous leprosy (295–296).

HISTOLOGY (FIGURE 9-5A–C):
■ **Indeterminate Leprosy:** It shows a superficial and deep perivascular, periadnexal, and perineurial infiltrate composed predominantly of lymphocytes with rare macrophages. Bacteria are difficult to find, and when present they can be seen around nerves.
■ "Recently it has been reported that there are two species of M. leprae, with the newly described one being responsible for lepromatous leprosy." (Han et al) [from MD Anderson CC]
■ **Tuberculoid Leprosy:** It shows well-formed linear epithelioid granulomas in dermis that often display perineurial inflammation. The granulomas have many Langhans cells and are surrounded by lymphocytes. Granulomas may erode the undersurface of the epidermis. Dermal nerves can be fragmented due to the granulomas. S100 immunostain may be helpful in identifying nerve fragmentation. Chronic inflammatory response around the eccrine glands is commonly seen. Bacilli are rarely identified.
■ **Borderline Tuberculoid Leprosy:** It shows epithelioid cell granulomas but few or no lymphocytes or Langhans giant cells as seen in tuberculoid leprosy. Bacilli are absent or rare.
■ **Borderline Leprosy:** It shows many epithelioid histiocytes without the formation of well-defined granulomas. A grenz zone is readily seen. Langhans giant cells are minimal and lymphocytes are more dispersed. Bacilli are rarely identified.
■ **Borderline Lepromatous Leprosy:** It shows collections of large macrophages with abundant granular cytoplasm (some may have foamy cytoplasm). Lymphocytes are present, and some are associated with dermal nerves. Nerves may have an onion-skin appearance and a grenz zone is present. Bacilli are easily identified.
■ **Lepromatous Leprosy:** It shows sheets of foamy macrophages within the dermis with minimal lymphocytic infiltrate and a noticeable grenz zone. Subcutaneous and deep dermal inflammatory nodules are rarely present. There are numerous acid-fast bacilli seen within the foamy macrophages. The macrophages usually express S100p.
■ **Histoid Leprosy:** It is a variant of lepromatous leprosy with a diffuse fascicular arrangement of spindled cells in the dermis admixed with foamy macrophages. Some cases may resemble a dermatofibroma. Numerous bacilli are readily identified.
■ Mycobacterium leprae is best demonstrated by modifications of the Ziehl–Neelsen stain, such as the Fite stain.

Leprosy

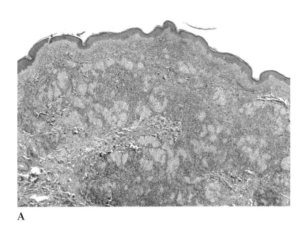

A

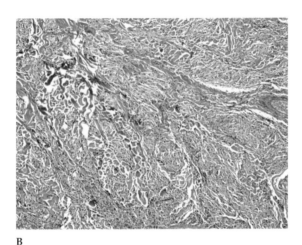

B

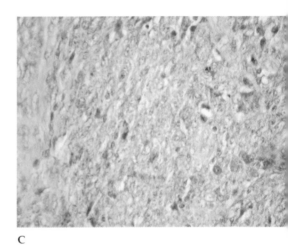

C

FIGURE 9-5 *Tuberculoid Leprosy*
A. Naked granulomas surrounded by a dense lymphocytic infiltrate. **B.** *Lepromatous Leprosy.* Dense histiocytic infiltrate in dermis. Note the macrophages have large abundant granular cytoplasm. **C.** Fite stain showing many acid-fast bacilli.

Syphilis

Syphilis is caused by *Treponema pallidum* and represents a chronic venereal disease with multiple clinical presentations. It is divided into primary, secondary, latent, and tertiary stages. The primary lesion is a superficial ulcer (chancre) in the area of contact. The chancre is an indurated, painless ulcer that appears approximately 21 days after sexual exposure. Secondary syphilis usually manifests 3–12 weeks after the appearance of a chancre as maculopapular or erythematosquamous lesions on the skin. More than 95% of patients with secondary syphilis show cutaneous lesions on the palms and soles that evolve to become annular or papulosquamous. Genital lesions include condyloma lata (papillomatous whitish plaques). Screening tests include the RPR test and the VDRL test; sensitivities are 80% for primary syphilis and approach 100% for secondary syphilis, although they can yield high false-positive rates. The FTA-ABS test is reactive in 85% of primary syphilis cases, 99–100% of secondary syphilis cases, and 95% of latent or late syphilis cases. Some concomitant diseases, such as AIDS, may result in false negative results (298, 299).

HISTOLOGY (FIGURE 9-6A, B):
- **Primary Syphilis:** It shows epidermal necrosis, diffuse lymphoplasmacytic infiltrate in dermis, and endothelial swelling and proliferation. The treponemas can usually be visualized by Warthin–Starry stains. Dark-field examination of a smear from a chancre will readily show the spirochete.
- **Secondary Syphilis:** It shows a superficial and deep perivascular infiltrate usually composed of lymphocytes and variable number of plasma cells. The dermal blood vessels are dilated and thickened, and are lined by plump endothelial cells. The epidermis shows psoriasiform hyperplasia and mild spongiotic changes. The dermal-epidermal junction is often infiltrated by lymphocytes. There may be a lichenoid lymphoplasmacytic infiltrate and granulomas, especially in older lesions. There may be plasma cells in the perineurium. Silver stains such as Warthin–Starry may reveal the spirochetes; however, immunohistochemistry is more sensitive for detecting *Treponema pallidum* in tissue.

Syphilis

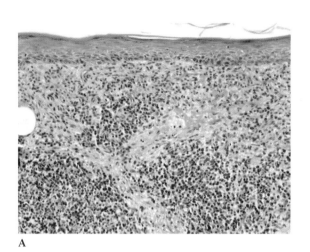 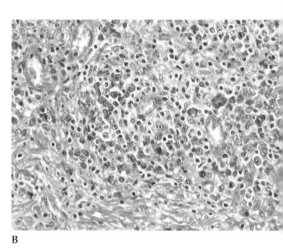

A   B

FIGURE 9-6 *Secondary Syphilis*
A. Dense lichenoid and superficial perivascular lymphoplasmacytic infiltrate.
B. Higher magnification shows a dense lymphoplasmacytic infiltrate.

Lyme Disease (Erythema Chronicum Migrans)

Lyme disease is an infection caused by the spirochete *Borrelia burgdorferi*, and is transmitted from host to host by the Ixodes, or deer tick. The cutaneous lesion in Lyme disease, known as erythema chronicum migrans, is a centrifugally spreading annular erythematous lesion at the site of the bite of the tick. In some patients extracutaneous signs can be seen including arthritis, nerve palsies, carditis, meningitis, etc. (300, 301).

HISTOLOGY (FIGURE 9-7A, B):
- Superficial and deep perivascular and interstitial inflammatory infiltrate (mainly composed of lymphocytes, plasma cells, and eosinophils)
- The inflammatory response can be seen extending into the subcutaneous fat.
- Endothelial cell swelling
- The epidermis may show mild spongiosis, exocytosis, and apoptotic cells.
- The bacteria can be found by Warthin–Starry stain near the dermoepidermal junction and in superficial dermis.

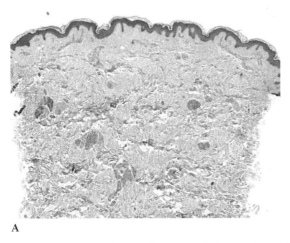
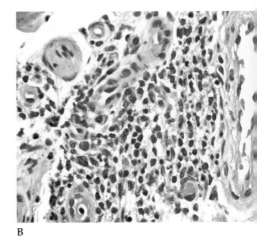

A   B

FIGURE 9-7 *Erythema Chronicum Migrans (ECM)*
A. The biopsy shows a superficial and deep lymphocytic infiltrate in a tight perivascular arrangement. The infiltrate is composed of lymphocytes, histiocytes and rare plasma cells and eosinophils. **B.** High power magnification showing scattered plasma cells around perivascular spaces. The presence of plasma cells and eosinophils favors ECM over other forms of gyrate erythema.

Bacillary Angiomatosis

Bacillary angiomatosis is caused by two gram-negative coccobacilli, *Bartonella henselae* and *Bartonella quintana*. Bacillary angiomatosis can affect almost any organ system, although it most commonly affects skin and subcutaneous tissue. It is most commonly seen in patients with HIV infection, but has also been reported in patients with leukemia, immunocompromised patients, and in organ transplant. Cutaneous lesions are usually multiple and take the form of pyogenic granuloma-like lesions, subcutaneous nodules, and hyperpigmented indurated plaques, typically on extremities (302–304).

HISTOLOGY:
- Small round blood vessels in an edematous dermal stroma
- The vessels show plump cuboidal epithelioid endothelial cells.
- The inflammatory response is composed of lymphocytes, histiocytes, and neutrophils.
- Characteristic clumps of granular purple material, which represent the organisms
- Usually epidermal collarette and ulceration (especially in superficial lesions)
- The organisms can be easily seen using Giemsa or Warthin–Starry stain.

DIFFERENTIAL DIAGNOSIS:
- The main differential diagnosis is with Kaposi sarcoma; however, the presence of neutrophils, epithelioid endothelial cells, and clumps of granular purple material is characteristic of bacillary angiomatosis.
- Pyogenic granulomas will show also similar features and are sometimes impossible to distinguish them until bacteria are detected in the special stains in bacillary angiomatosis.

Dermatophytosis

Dermatophytosis is caused by a closely related group of fungi known as dermatophytes which have the ability to use keratin as a nutrient source. Clinically, they present with scaly, erythematous, and annular plaques. Three genera have been involved: *Trichophyton, Epidermophyton,* and *Microsporum* (305–309).

HISTOLOGY (FIGURE 9-8A, B):
- Wide range of histological changes.
- Most commonly compact orthokeratosis, sometimes as the "sandwich sign" (orthokeratosis or parakeratosis alternating in layers with basket-weave stratum corneum), and neutrophils in stratum corneum.
- The epidermis may show psoriasiform hyperplasia, mild spongiosis, microvesicle formation, subcorneal pustules, eosinophils, and spongiosis.
- In dermis perivascular infiltrate composed of lymphocytes, eosinophils, and neutrophils.
- Skin may appear normal.
- PAS stain should be considered in any inflammatory dermatosis with parakeratosis and neutrophils.

VARIANTS:
Tinea Capitis: More common in children, and clinically it presents with scale crust and broken hairs along sometimes with adenopathy and alopecia. The organisms may not be noted within the stratum corneum. Fungal spores may be localized within the hair shafts (endothrix) or around the hair surface (ectothrix). The most common implicated organism in United States is *T. tonsurans.* "Favus" is a severe form of tinea capitis that presents with prominent perifollicular hyperkeratotic crusts (scutula), usually caused by *T. schoenleinii* (**Figure 9-8C**).

Majocchi Granuloma: Nodular granulomatous perifolliculitis caused by rupture of an infected follicle. Lesions are most commonly seen in females and located in the lower extremity. It is mostly caused by *T. rubrum, M. canis,* or *T. violaceum* (**Figure 9-8D**).

Kerion: A severe inflammatory boggy plaque usually on the scalp. Caused mainly by *M. canis.*

Tinea Faciae: Tinea of the face, as a persistent eruption of red macules. Usually caused by *T. rubrum.*

Tinea Barbae: Tinea limited to the beard. Usually caused by *T. verrucosum.*

Tinea Corporis: Infection of the trunk and extremities, more common in adult males. Most commonly caused by *T. rubrum* followed by *M. canis.*

Tinea Cruris: Sharply demarcated erythematous patches in the groin area. It is usually caused by *T. rubrum*, but also associated with *T. mentagrophytes* and *E. floccosum.*

Tinea Manuum: Infection of the hands, usually associated with tinea pedis. Usually caused by *T. rubrum, E. floccosum,* or *T. mentagrophytes.*

Tinea Pedis: Tinea of the feet; clinically it may resemble contact dermatitis. Usually caused by *T. rubrum,* or *T. mentagrophytes.*

Tinea Unguium (Onychomycosis): Tinea of the nails, caused by any fungal organism including dermatophytes, Candida, etc. However, most cases are due to dermatophyte infections.

Dermatophytosis

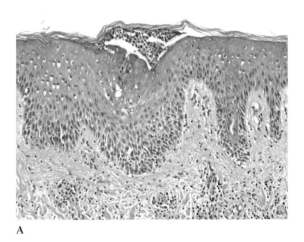

A

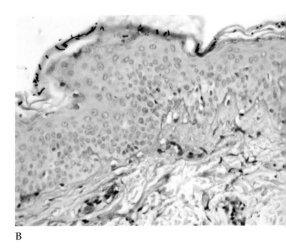

B

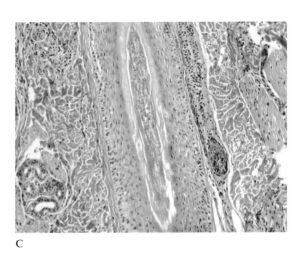

C

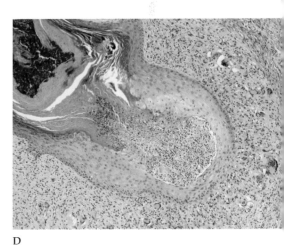

D

FIGURE 9-8 *Dermatophytosis*
A. Neutrophilic collection in stratum corneum. **B.** PAS stain showing many hyphae within stratum corneum. **C.** *Tinea Capitis.* Endothrix (fungal spores may be localized within the hair shafts). **D.** *Majocchi Granuloma.* Granulomatous perifolliculitis due to the presence of fungal organisms within the adventitial dermis around the infected follicle.

Tinea Versicolor

It is a benign, superficial cutaneous fungal infection that clinically is characterized by hypopigmented or hyperpigmented macules on the chest and the back. Tinea versicolor is caused by *Malassezia globosa* and *Malassezia furfur* (310, 311).

HISTOLOGY (FIGURE 9-9A, B):
- Mild epidermal spongiosis with a superficial perivascular lymphocytic infiltrate.
- In the stratum corneum there are numerous round budding yeasts and short septate hyphae mimicking the shapes of "spaghetti and meatballs".
- The organisms can be highlighted by PAS.

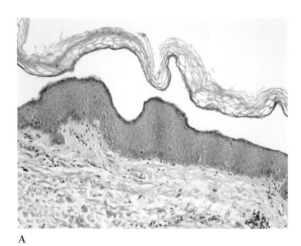

A

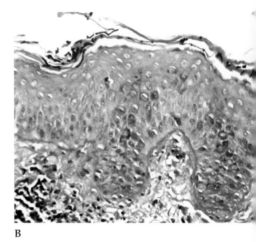

B

FIGURE 9-9 *Tinea Versicolor*
A. Epidermal acanthosis and spongiosis and a thickened stratum corneum with many hyphae. **B.** PAS stain showing the numerous round budding yeasts and short septate hyphae.

Tinea Nigra

Tinea nigra is a rare superficial fungal infection caused by a dematiaceous (pigmented) fungus, *Phaeoannellomyces werneckii*. Clinically, it presents as brown to black macules involving the palms or soles (312).

HISTOLOGY:
- The stratum corneum is mildly orthokeratotic.
- Multiple brown hyphae and spores are noted within the stratum corneum.
- The organisms can be highlighted by PAS.

Chromomycosis

Chromomycosis (chromoblastomycosis) is a chronic fungal infection that starts as a scaly nodule, caused by traumatic inoculation of a dematiaceous fungus (*Fonsecaea pedrosoi*, *Phialophora verrucosa*, *Cladosporium carrionii*). Squamous cell carcinoma may be associated with chromomycosis (313, 314).

HISTOLOGY (FIGURE 9-10):
■ Pseudoepitheliomatous hyperplasia of the epidermis
■ Intraepidermal microabscesses
■ Diffuse granulomatous and lymphocytic inflammatory infiltrate in dermis (occasional eosinophils)
■ Round, thick-walled (cigar shaped), golden brown cells (sclerotic bodies) can be seen in giant cells and within the intraepidermal microabscesses by H&E stains.

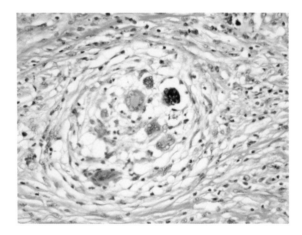

FIGURE 9-10 *Chromomycosis (Chromoblastomycosis)* Characteristic round, thick-walled golden brown cells (sclerotic bodies).

Phaeohyphomycosis

Phaeohyphomycosis includes a diverse group of dematiaceous fungal infections that are seen in immunocompromised patients, commonly after trauma with implantation of a wood splinter or other vegetable matter. Different categories have been described including the superficial (black "piedra"), cutaneous, subcutaneous, and systemic type. The most commonly associated fungi in cutaneous and subcutaneous lesions are *Exophiala jeanselmei* and *Wangiella dermatitidis* (315).

HISTOLOGY:
- Cystic lesion or abscess located in deep dermis and subcutaneous fat
- Granulomatous reaction in the wall of the lesion fibrous tissue
- Central cystic space containing necrotic debris
- Occasionally wood splinter
- Brown filamentous hyphae and yeast-like structures in the wall, giant cells, and/or in the debris

Sporotrichosis

Sporotrichosis is a subcutaneous or systemic infection caused by *Sporothrix schenckii* (dimorphic fungus). Cutaneous infection often results from a puncture wound involving rose thorns or wood splinters. The characteristic infection involves suppurative subcutaneous nodules that progress proximally along lymphatic channels (316–318).

HISTOLOGY:
- The epidermis shows pseudoepitheliomatous hyperplasia.
- Granulomatous inflammatory response with suppuration in the dermis.
- The organisms can be demonstrated as yeast, "cigar" bodies, or hyphae.
- Characteristic sporotrix asteroid body (yeast form surrounded by intensely eosinophilic, ray-like processes).

Cryptococcosis

Cryptococcosis is an infection caused by the encapsulated yeast *Cryptococcus neoformans* (dimorphic fungus). The primary site of infection is most often the lungs; however, the disease frequently manifests with signs of extrapulmonary dissemination, involving the skin in approximately 13% of cases. Most patients are immunocompromised and this infection is a well-known occurrence in patients with AIDS (319, 320).

HISTOLOGY (FIGURE 9-11):
- The infection may show tuberculoid granulomas in the dermis and subcutis, with only few organisms.
- Sometimes the lesion may show large numbers of organisms in a foamy stroma with little or no inflammation.
- The organisms are oval, thick-walled spherules surrounded by a polysaccharide capsule.
- Special stains, such as mucicarmine, will highlight the capsule.
- Organisms with thin capsule ("capsule deficient") may be associated with more aggressive behavior.

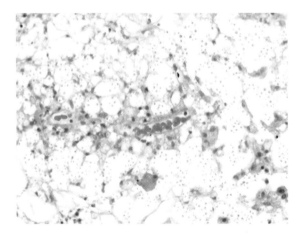

FIGURE 9-11 *Cryptococcosis*
Many organisms with oval, thick-walled spherules surrounded by an empty space, the polysaccharide capsule.

Fusariosis

It is a hyalohyphomycosis caused by *Fusarium sp* and can produce a localized cutaneous lesion or disseminated disease. Systemic disease is mainly seen in immunocompromised patients with hematological malignancies (321, 322).

HISTOLOGY (FIGURE 9-12):
- The reaction in dermis is mainly composed of a dense acute and chronic inflammatory response that may involve the subcutaneous fat.
- Dermal necrosis with vascular thrombosis
- The hyphae are hyaline, septate, and branched at multiple angles. Dilated conidiophores at the end of the hyphae ("ice cream" appearance).

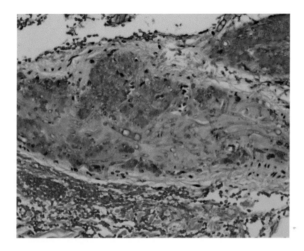

FIGURE 9-12 *Fusariosis*
Hyphae are hyaline, septate, and branched at multiple angles. Characteristic dilated conidiophores at the end of the hyphae (ice-cream appearance).

Coccidiomycosis

Coccidiomycosis is caused by *Coccidioides immitis* (dimorphic fungus). It is endemic to the Southwestern United States and in Central America and South America. Most commonly it presents as an acute self-limited pulmonary infection resulting from inhalation of the arthrospores. Rarely, in immunocompromised patients dissemination may happen, and the skin may be affected showing a verrucous lesion usually on the face (nasolabial area) (323–325).

HISTOLOGY (FIGURE 9-13):
- ◼ Pseudoepitheliomatous hyperplasia of the epidermis
- ◼ Noncaseating granulomas in the dermis
- ◼ The organisms show thick-walled spherules with endospores in H&E stains (present within the granulomas, often within the multinucleate giant cells).

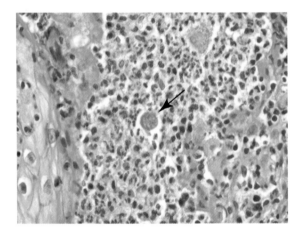

FIGURE 9-13 *Coccidiomycosis*
Organisms show thick-walled spherules with endospores.

Blastomycosis

Blastomycosis is caused by *Blastomyces dermatitidis* (dimorphic fungus). It is endemic in Mississippi, Missouri, Ohio River, and the Great Lakes. Infection occurs by inhalation of the conidial forms of the fungus from its natural soil habitat. The skin is the most common site of extrapulmonary blastomycosis and is involved in about 20–40% of the cases (326, 327).

HISTOLOGY (FIGURE 9-14A, B):
- Pseudoepitheliomatous hyperplasia
- Polymorphous dermal infiltrate composed of lymphocytes, histiocytes, and neutrophils with scattered giant cells
- Microabscesses are characteristically seen in the dermis and in the acanthotic epidermis.
- Granulomas and suppurative granulomas
- The yeast forms are best visualized with a PAS stain.
- The organisms are thick-walled broad-based budding yeasts present extracellularly in the dermis or intracellularly in multinucleated giant cells.
- Demonstration of the yeasts is particularly important in blastomycosis since the pseudoepitheliomatous hyperplasia observed in the tissue may simulate squamous cell carcinoma.
- The hyperplastic epidermis lacks the cytological atypia of squamous cell carcinoma.

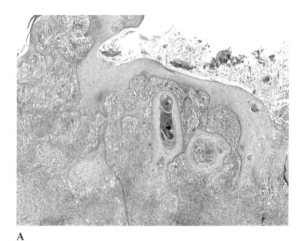
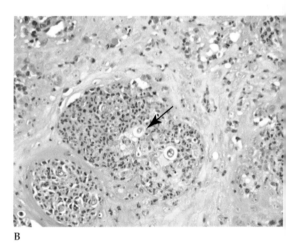

A   B

FIGURE 9-14 *Blastomycosis*
A. Pseudoepitheliomatous hyperplasia with a polymorphous dermal infiltrate with characteristic neutrophilic microabscesses within epidermis. **B.** High power reveals thick-walled, broad-based budding yeasts within the neutrophilic microabscesses.

Histoplasmosis

Histoplasmosis is caused by *Histoplasma capsulatum* (dimorphic fungus). It is endemic to the Ohio, Missouri, and Mississippi River valleys. The infection is acquired by the inhalation of spores from soil contaminated by bird and bat droppings. The lung is the most common primary focus of involvement and most patients are asymptomatic; those who develop clinical manifestations are usually immunocompromised. Cutaneous lesions are rare and can be primary or secondary to the pulmonary infection (328–330).

HISTOLOGY (FIGURE 9-15):
■ Changes are mainly seen in dermis as a granulomatous inflammatory response, occasionally extending into the subcutaneous fat.
■ Numerous parasitized macrophages containing small ovoid yeast-like organisms with a clear halo.
■ GMS stain highlights the organisms.

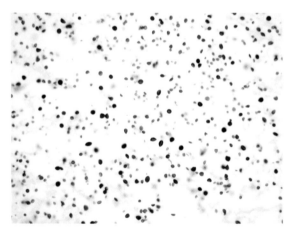

FIGURE 9-15 *Histoplasmosis*
GMS highlighting the numerous parasitized macrophages (ovoid yeast-like organisms with a clear halo).

Paracoccidioidomycosis

Paracoccidioidomycosis is caused by *Paracoccidioides brasiliensis* (dimorphic fungus). It is endemic to South and Central America. Most commonly presents as a chronic progressive systemic mycosis with pulmonary infection as the most common manifestation; however, following dissemination, it may involve the mucous membranes, skin, and lymph nodes (331, 332).

HISTOLOGY (FIGURE 9-16):
- Pseudoepitheliomatous hyperplasia
- Acute and chronic inflammatory response admixed with granulomas in dermis
- Characteristic small and large thick wall budding yeasts with a double-contour and with buds distributed on the surface in a steering-wheel appearance
- The organisms can be found in the giant cells and lying free in the tissue.
- The organisms are best highlighted with GMS.

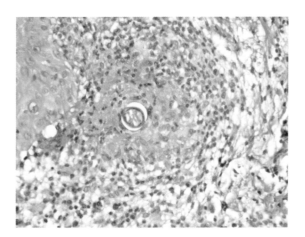

FIGURE 9-16 *Paracoccidiomycosis*
Characteristic large thick wall budding yeasts with a double-contour and with buds distributed on the surface (steering-wheel appearance).

Zygomycosis

Zygomycosis is a broad term to refer to an infection including mucormycosis, phyco-mycosis, and basidiobolomycosis. We will mainly refer to mucormycosis since they are the most commonly seen in humans. Mucormycosis is an opportunistic infection by fungi within the family Mucoraceae. There are three main genera responsible for human infections: *Rhizopus*, *Mucor*, and *Absidia*. Primary cutaneous mucormycosis is rare and usually develops in diabetes, leukemia, neutropenia, etc. Secondary cutaneous mucormycosis results from hematogenous seeding (333, 334).

HISTOLOGY (FIGURE 9-17)
■ The histology can be quite variable ranging from minimal inflammatory response to massive areas of suppuration and necrosis.
■ The hyphae are broad, lack septa, and they branch at 90-degree angles, as opposed to Aspergillus, which branches at an acute angle.
■ The hyphae often invade the vessel walls with subsequent thrombosis and infarction.
■ The hyphae are identified by H&E, PAS, and methenamine silver stains.

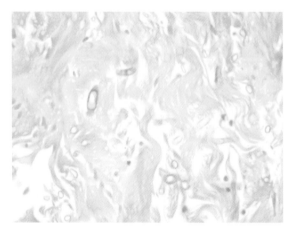

FIGURE 9-17 *Zygomycosis*
Hyphae are broad, lack septa, and they branch at 90-degree angles (mucormycosis).

Aspergillosis

Aspergillosis is one of the most common opportunistic infections seen in immuno-compromised patients mainly affecting the pulmonary system; however, it may rarely involve the skin. *Aspergillus fumigatus* is the most common human pathogen, followed by *A. flavus*, *A. niger*, and *A. terreus*. Cutaneous aspergillosis can arise as a primary infection or secondary to disseminated disease. *A. fumigatus* is most commonly associated with disseminated disease with cutaneous involvement and *A. flavus* least frequently causes primary cutaneous infection (335–337).

HISTOLOGY (FIGURE 9-18A, B):
- Variable granulomatous to neutrophilic inflammatory response.
- Narrow septated hyphae that branch at an acute angle.
- When numerous, hyphae arrange parallel to each other.
- In disseminated disease, the hyphae may invade the walls of dermal blood vessels producing thrombosis and some associated necrosis.
- The hyphae are best shown by silver methenamine or PAS stain.

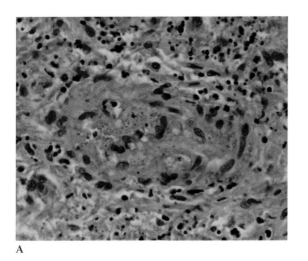
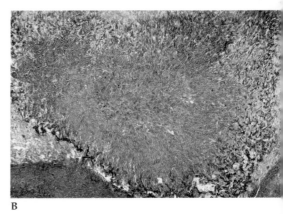

A   B

FIGURE 9-18 *Aspergillosis*
A. Numerous, narrow, and septated hyphae invading blood vessels. **B.** Silver methenamine showing many narrow septated hyphae that branch at acute angle.

Rhinosporidiosis

It is a chronic granulomatous infection of the mucocutaneous tissue that clinically manifests as polypoid pedunculated nodules that arise from the nasal mucosa or external structures of the eye. It is caused by the hydrophilic agent *Rhinosporidium seeberi*, which was initially regarded as a fungus, but now by molecular biological techniques has been demonstrated to be a parasite. Cutaneous infection is rare and autoinoculation is more common than primary cutaneous origin (338, 339).

HISTOLOGY (FIGURE 9-19):
- Epithelial acanthosis with slight hyperkeratosis
- Large spherical sporangia containing from hundreds of endospores in submucosa
- The sporangia are free in tissue or may be within the giant cells.
- Submucosal mixed inflammatory cell infiltrate with the formation of some granulomas

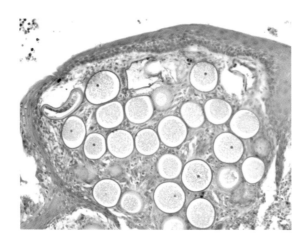

FIGURE 9-19 *Rhinosporidiosis*
Large spherical sporangia containing from hundreds of endospores in submucosa.

Lobomycosis

Lobomycosis, also known as keloidal blastomycosis, is a self-limited, chronic fungal infection of the skin endemic in rural regions in South America near the Amazon/ Orinoco rivers. The disease is caused by *Loboa loboi*; but based on recent molecular studies, *Lacazia loboi* is the current recommended name. Clinically, it presents as slow growing keloidal plaques and nodules (340–342).

PATHOLOGY (FIGURE 9-20):
- Acanthotic or hyperplastic epidermis
- Granulomatous inflammatory response in deep dermis and subcutis
- The granulomas have many histiocytes, multinucleated giant cells, asteroid bodies.
- Numerous round fungi with transparent cytoplasm and a double thick wall are lined up in rows (forming beads joined by a thin bridge).

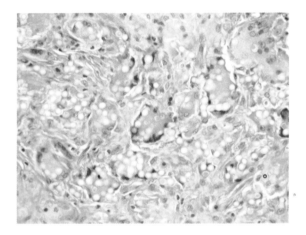

FIGURE 9-20 *Lobomycosis*
Numerous round to oval fungi with transparent cytoplasm and a double thick wall lined up in rows (forming beads joined by a thin bridge).

Human Papillomavirus Infection (Warts)

Human papillomavirus (HPV) is a papovavirus (double stranded DNA virus) and is one of the most common viral infections in humans. HPV is transmitted by direct or indirect contact. The primary clinical manifestations of HPV infection include common warts, genital warts, and deep palmoplantar warts. Many types of HPV have been identified. Common warts: HPV types 2 and 4 (most common); palmoplantar warts (myrmecia): HPV type 1 (most common) and HPV 4; flat warts: HPV types 3, 10, and 28; butcher warts: HPV type 7; focal epithelial hyperplasia (Heck disease): HPV types 13 and 32; Cystic warts: HPV type 60; epidermodysplasia verruciformis (EDV): most common HPV 3 and 5; condyloma accuminatum: HPV 6, 8, 11, 16, and 18 (343–348).

HISTOLOGY (FIGURE 9-21A, B):

- **Common Warts (Verruca Vulgaris):** Marked hyperkeratosis and papillomatosis with often some inward growth of the elongated rete ridges at the edge of the lesion. Columns of parakeratosis with small deposits of hemorrhage and the presence of large vacuolated cells (koilocytes) in upper epidermis and in the granular layer.
- **Flat Wart (Verruca Plana):** Basket weave hyperkeratosis without papillomatosis. Characteristic vacuolation of the granular and upper epidermis.
- **Condyloma Accuminatum:** Polypoid configuration with marked acanthosis, with focal papillomatosis and hyperkeratosis. Vacuolization of granular cells is not as marked as in verruca vulgaris. Some lesions resemble seborrheic keratosis.
- **Epidermodysplasia Verruciformis (EDV):** Some lesions may resemble flat warts but the keratinocytes are large and sometimes arranged in nests, in the granular and spinous layers. There is a conspicuous perinuclear halo and the cytoplasm is blue-gray in color and contains keratohyaline granules of various sizes and shapes (**Figure 9-21C**).
- **Focal Epithelial Hyperplasia (Hecks Disease):** Most commonly seen in the mucosa of the lips and cheeks. The epithelium is usually hyperplastic, acanthotic and with some elongation of the rete ridges. The epidermal cells are pale, particularly in the upper layers, and sometimes they can show binucleation.

Human Papillomavirus Infection (Warts)

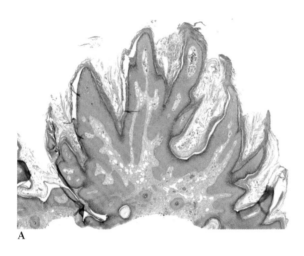

A

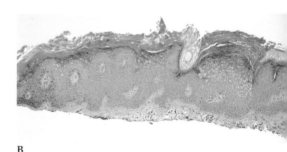

B

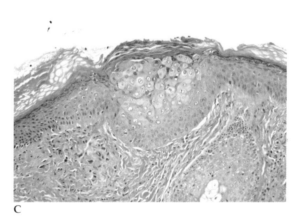

C

FIGURE 9-21
A. *Verruca Vulgaris.* Hyperkeratosis and papillomatosis with focal inward growth of the elongated rete ridges at the edges. Note the presence of large vacuolated cells (koilocytes) in upper epidermis and in the granular layer. **B.** *Flat Wart.* Basket weave hyperkeratosis without papillomatosis and HPV changes in the granular layer **C.** *Epidermodysplasia verruciformis (EDV).* Large keratinocytes with blue cytoplasm are characteristic of EDV. However, keratinocytes with similar morphology may be seen as an incidental finding in other cutaneous lesions such as actinic and seborrheic keratosis.

Herpes Infections

Herpes simplex virus (HSV) infection is a common mucocutaneous disease characterized by grouped vesicles on an erythematous base. There are two types of HSV, HSV type 1 and HSV type 2. HSV-1, known as a "cold sore," is characterized by the presence of vesicles usually in the lips but may affect the oral cavity, pharynx, etc. HSV-1 is transmitted through direct contact with infected saliva or with contaminated utensils. HSV type 2 infection generally involves the genitalia and surrounding areas after puberty; it is usually sexually transmitted. HSV-2 in children may be an indication of child abuse (349, 350).

Chickenpox (varicella) is caused by the varicella zoster virus (VZV) and is a highly contagious disease. The incubation period is of 11 to 20 days, then varicella results in a widespread vesicular eruption on the face and trunk. Most patients are children, although infection is occasionally seen in adults, and then associated with increased morbidity and even death (351, 352).

Herpes zoster (shingles) is a common cutaneous infection that results from reactivation of latent VZV infection. It has an increased incidence in the elderly, and in those who are immunocompromised.

HISTOLOGY (FIGURE 9-22A, B):
■ Herpes virus infections show similar histomorphology.
■ Epidermal acantholysis with several multinucleated keratinocytes with glassy intranuclear inclusions (Cowdry type A)
■ Dense lymphocytic infiltrate in the dermis along with lymphocytic vasculitis
■ Perineural lymphocytic infiltrate
■ Immunohistochemical studies against either Herpes subtype may help detecting the infected cells both in the epithelium and also other dermal structures (e.g., infected vessels).

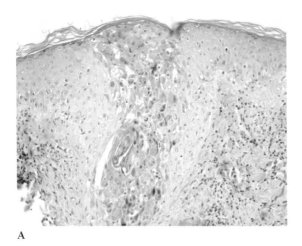 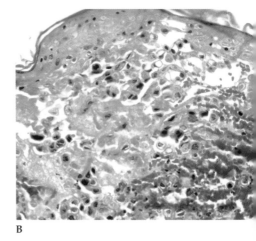

A   B

FIGURE 9-22 *Herpes*
A. Herpes involving the hair follicle (Zoster), and showing multinucleated keratinocytes with molding. **B.** Intraepidermal acantholysis with several multinucleated keratinocytes with glassy intranuclear inclusions.

Molluscum Contagiosum

Molluscum contagiosum is a cutaneous infection caused by a large brick-shaped DNA poxvirus. Transmission of molluscum contagiosum has been reported by direct skin contact. Molluscum contagiosum occurs as solitary or multiple dome-shaped, umbilicated, waxy papules. There is a predilection for the head and neck, trunk, or the genitalia of children and adolescents (353, 354).

HISTOLOGY (FIGURE 9-23A, B):
- Inverted lobules of acanthotic and hyperplastic epidermis
- Eosinophilic inclusion bodies form in the cytoplasm of keratinocytes just above the basal layer (Henderson-Patterson or molluscum bodies).
- The viral bodies increase in size as they progress up toward the granular layer causing compression of the nucleus to the periphery of the infected keratinocytes.

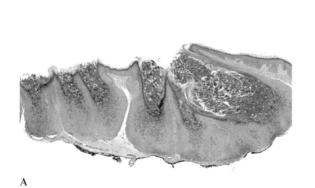 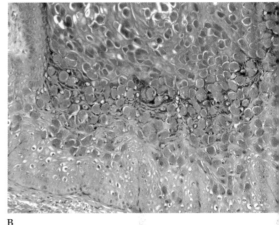

A   B

FIGURE 9-23 *Molluscum Contagiosum*
A. Inverted lobules of acanthotic and hyperplastic epidermis with characteristic eosinophilic inclusion bodies in the cytoplasm of keratinocytes. **B.** Higher magnification of the eosinophilic inclusion bodies in the cytoplasm of keratinocytes (Henderson-Patterson bodies).

Orf and Milker Nodule

Orf (ecthyma contagiosum) is primarily a disease of sheep and goats and it is caused by a poxvirus of the paravaccinia subgroup. Orf can be transmitted to humans by contact with infected animals. Lesions are firm red papules that develop most commonly on the hands and forearms. Spontaneous regression eventually occurs by 3–6 weeks (355–357).

   Milker nodule is also caused by a poxvirus and produces mild infections of the teats and mouths of cows. The lesions affect the hands of dairy farmers and the incubation period is of 5 days to 2 weeks. The lesions are usually multiple (358, 359).

HISTOLOGY:
- **Orf:** The lesion shows epidermal acanthosis with marked intercellular and intracellular edema, vacuolization, and ballooning degeneration. Cytoplasmic inclusion bodies are usually present. The superficial dermis contains a dense inflammatory infiltrate of plasma cells, macrophages, histiocytes, lymphocytes, and prominent vascularity (sometimes with simulating a vascular tumor). Late lesions may show central epidermal necrosis.
- **Milker Nodule:** In the early stage, the lesion shows vacuolization and ballooning degeneration of the cells in upper epidermis with intraepidermal microvesicles. There are common intracytoplasmic inclusions (rarely intranuclear inclusions too). Epidermal necrosis can be seen. In the late stage, the lesion shows acanthosis and hyperplasia of the epidermis along with edema of the papillary dermis. Also, there is an inflammatory response composed of lymphocytes, histiocytes, plasma cells, and rare eosinophils. A vascular proliferation is usually present in superficial dermis.

Gianotti-Crosti Syndrome
(Papular Acrodermatitis of Childhood)

Gianotti-Crosti syndrome (GCS) is a distinct self-limited disease characterized by an erythematous eruption, lymphadenopathy and acute anicteric hepatitis. The skin lesions appear as multiple non-pruritic, flat-topped erythematous papules located mainly in the head and neck area and extremities (torso is usually spared). This dermatosis most likely represents a type IV hypersensitivity reaction to viral or bacterial organisms. Hepatitis B has been commonly associated; however, other viruses such as Epstein-Barr virus, enterovirus, cytomegalovirus, hepatitis A, etc., have been also associated with this disorder (360–362).

HISTOLOGY:
- Epidermal spongiosis with exocytosis (pityriasiform spongiosis)
- Mild vacuolar interface damage
- Dense tight perivascular lymphocytic infiltrate with endothelial cell swelling (true vasculitis is not seen)
- Mild papillary edema

Lymphogranuloma Venereum

Lymphogranuloma venereum (LGV) is a sexually transmitted disease that is caused by serovars L1, L2, and L3 of Chlamydia trachomatis. The clinical manifestations of LGV vary depending on the disease stage and are divided into primary, secondary, and tertiary stages. The primary stage presents as a small papule or ulcer on the genital area. The secondary stage presents with regional painful lymphadenopathy (lymph nodes may rupture). Constitutional symptoms are common at this stage. The tertiary stage, the chronic inflammatory reaction can lead to fistulas, strictures, rectal stenoses, and lymphedema (363, 364).

HISTOLOGY:
- Ulcerated lesions with granulomatous inflammation admixed with many plasma cells
- Endothelial cell swelling
- Giemsa stain may reveal the Chlamydia
- DIF (using a fluorescein-labeled antibody) detects C. trachomatis

Leishmaniasis

Leishmaniasis is a disease caused by the protozoa of the Leishmania species, which is transmitted by the bite of a female sandfly. Clinically, it can present in various ways, and is classified as: 1) cutaneous leishmaniasis (oriental) caused by *L. tropica* in Asia and Africa and by *L. mexicana* in Central and South America, 2) mucocutaneous leishmaniasis (American) caused by *L. braziliensis*, and 3) visceral leishmaniasis (kala-azar) caused by *L. donovani*. In cutaneous leishmaniasis, after the bite of an infected sandfly, the incubation period is usually several weeks after inoculation. Initially, the lesion is a small red papule that over several weeks becomes darker and crusts in the center, eventually ulcerating. There may be regional adenopathy, satellite lesions, and subcutaneous nodule. Mucocutaneous leishmaniasis can be the primary manifestation of the disease and the incubation period is from 1–3 months. Cutaneous lesions usually develop and the mucosal lesions often appear after the primary cutaneous lesion has resolved. Mucosal lesions can progress to involve the entire nasal mucosa (365–368).

HISTOLOGY (FIGURE 9-24):

■ **Cutaneous Leishmaniasis:** The biopsy shows an ulcerated epidermis with a diffuse dermal inflammatory response composed of lymphocytes, macrophages, giant cells, plasma cells, and sometimes a few eosinophils. The macrophages show many intracellular organisms that are round to oval basophilic structures and have an eccentrically located kinetoplast (amastigote forms "Leishman-Donovan" bodies) (the lack of a capsule is helpful in distinguishing them from Histoplasma). The organisms can be seen in H&E tissue sections but they are best seen on Giemsa stain (kinetoplast stains red).

■ Mucocutaneous leishmaniasis shows similar histology but with fewer organisms.

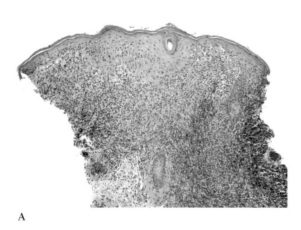 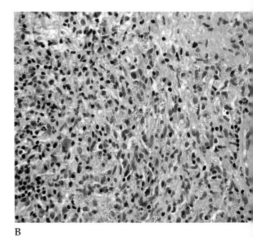

A   B

FIGURE 9-24 *Leishmaniasis*
A. The biopsy shows a diffuse dermal inflammatory response composed of histiocytes and lymphocytes. **B.** Characteristic macrophages showing many intracellular organisms that are round to oval basophilic and have an eccentrically located kinetoplast.

Amebiasis Cutis

Intestinal amebiasis is one of the most common causes of diarrhea in Central and South America and in other tropical areas. Amebiasis can cause cutaneous lesions (Amebiasis cutis) and is usually due to Entamoeba histolytica. Cutaneous lesion can be seen more commonly around the perianal area, but other sites can be affected as abdomen, buttocks, legs, etc. (369).

HISTOLOGY:

■ Trophozoites of E. histolytica are more likely found within the ulcer (12-20 μm).
■ Organisms are surrounded by lymphocytes and neutrophils.
■ Organisms frequently contain phagocytized red blood cells.
■ PAS stain highlights the organisms.

Protothecosis

Protothecosis is a rare exogenous infection caused by an achlorophyllic alga-like organism of the genus Prototheca, and the most common species in humans is *P. wickerhamii*. The skin is most commonly involved from primary inoculation through a wound or abrasion. The infection is usually localized; however, in immunocompromised patients, it can become widespread (370–372).

HISTOLOGY:
- Epidermis can be ulcerated.
- Granulomatous inflammatory response in dermis admixed with lymphocytes, plasma cells, eosinophils, and neutrophils.
- Areas of necrosis are common.
- Organisms (sporangia) are found in the cytoplasm of macrophages and multinucleate giant cells as thick-walled spherical bodies (septation and morula formation).
- Organisms are difficult to identify on H&E tissue sections and stain well with GMS and PAS.

Cysticercosis

Cysticercosis is a systemic disease caused by the larval form of the pork tapeworm, *Taenia solium*. Encystment of larvae can occur in almost any tissue and the most clinically important manifestation of the disease is involvement of the central nervous system (neurocysticercosis). On the skin, it presents as one or multiple asymptomatic subcutaneous nodules more commonly located on the chest and upper and lower extremities. Grossly, the nodules have a white cystic structure with an outer membrane containing clear fluid and a cysticercus larva at the periphery (373, 374).

HISTOLOGY (FIGURE 9-25):
- ◼ The cysticercus is surrounded by a cystic cavity.
- ◼ The scolex of the cysticercus larva is quite characteristic (hooklets and sucker caps).
- ◼ The cystic cavity is surrounded by a fibrous reaction with moderate chronic inflammatory response admixed with some eosinophils.
- ◼ Scattered giant cells

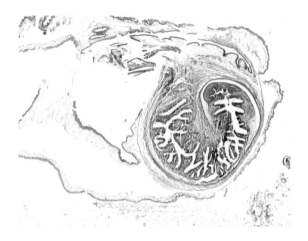

FIGURE 9-25 *Cysticercosis*
Scolex with characteristic hooklets and sucker caps.

Dirofilariasis

Human dirofilariasis clinically manifests as either subcutaneous nodules or lung parenchymal disease and in many cases asymptomatically. Infection with Dirofilaria is endemic in the Mediterranean region. The subcutaneous nodules are caused by Dirofilaria repens and the pulmonary disease is caused by *Dirofilaria immitis* (the dog heartworm) (375–378).

HISTOLOGY (FIGURE 9-26):
- Seen in subcutaneous tissue
- Degenerating filaria (coiled worm) with a laminated cuticle, longitudinal ridges, and large lateral chords is seen in the center of the nodule.
- Prominent inflammatory response composed of lymphocytes, plasma cells, histiocytes, eosinophils, and sometimes giant cells

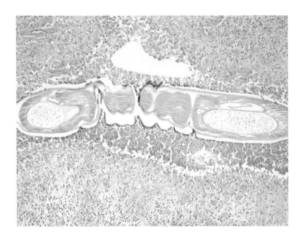

FIGURE 9-26 *Dirofilariasis*
Filaria (coiled worm) with a laminated cuticle and longitudinal ridges.

Onchocerciasis

The parasite, Onchocerca volvulus, is a nematode that belongs to the family *Filariidae*. *O. volvulus* is the only Onchocerca with a human host. Blackflies of the genus *Simulium* are the only vectors of O. volvulus. The classic lesion presents as a firm, painless nodule in the subcutaneous tissue (onchocercoma), in which the adult nematodes live and produce microfilariae. Cutaneous onchocerciasis (onchodermatitis) causes pruritus, a papular rash, scarring, and lichenification (leopard skin) (379–381).

HISTOLOGY (FIGURE 9-27):
- The subcutaneous nodules have an outer wall of dense fibrous tissue which usually extends between the worms.
- Within the nodule the adult worms have paired uteri.
- Centrally, there is granulation tissue with some calcification and foreign-body giant cells and a chronic inflammatory cell infiltrate with eosinophils.
- Microfilariae may be seen in lymphatics or lying free in dermis.

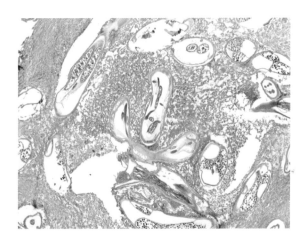

FIGURE 9-27 *Onchocerciasis*
Characteristic microfilariae seen lying free in dermis.

Cutaneous Larva Migrans

Cutaneous larva migrans (CLM) is most commonly found in tropical and subtropical geographic areas of the world. Clinically, CLM manifests as an erythematous and serpiginous cutaneous eruption caused by accidental percutaneous penetration and subsequent migration of larvae. The lesions are typically located on the dorsa of the feet and toes, anogenital region, the buttocks, the hands, and knees. CLM is most commonly caused by larvae of *Ancylostoma braziliense* (hookworm of wild and domestic dogs and cats), but *Necator americanus, Ancylostoma caninum, Uncinaria stenocephala,* and *Bunostomum phlebotomum* are other causes (382, 383).

HISTOLOGY (FIGURE 9-28):
■ Small burrows in the suprabasilar epidermis corresponding to the track of the larva (the parasite itself is rarely seen in tissue sections).
■ The epidermis also shows spongiosis with microvesicles formation, necrotic keratinocytes, and many eosinophils.
■ Dermis shows a superficial perivascular lymphocytic infiltrate admixed with eosinophils.

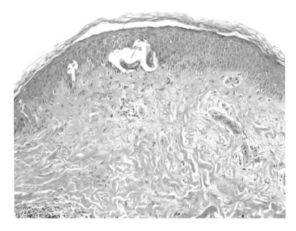

FIGURE 9-28 *Cutaneous Larva Migrans*
Small burrows in the suprabasilar epidermis
with parasite.

Scabies

Scabies is an intensely pruritic skin infestation caused by Sarcoptes scabiei var. hominis. Scabies is a great clinical imitator and its spectrum of cutaneous manifestations and associated symptoms often results in delayed diagnosis. Clinically, the primary lesion presents as small papules, vesicles, and burrows (axilla, groin, genitals, finger webs, etc.). The secondary lesions result from rubbing and scratching and they may be the only clinical manifestation of the disease. Nodular scabies is more common in children and young adults and presents as red pruritic nodules often on the penis and scrotum. Mites are rarely seen in this form and it is thought to represent a delayed hypersensitivity reaction. Norwegian (crusted) scabies is rare and contagious, and consists of widespread crusted and secondarily infected hyperkeratotic lesions, usually seen in physically debilitated and immunocompromised patients (urge to scratch) (384–386).

HISTOLOGY (FIGURE 9-29):
- Eggs, larvae, mites, and scybala (feces) in the stratum corneum
- Spongiosis and microvesicular formation with eosinophils and neutrophils
- Superficial and deep infiltrate of lymphocytes, histiocytes, and eosinophils
- **Nodular Scabies:** Shows a superficial and deep dense dermal inflammatory cell infiltrate composed of lymphocytes, histiocytes, plasma cells, and eosinophils. Lymphoid follicles can be seen and the infiltrate may extend into the subcutaneous fat. Mites are rarely found (20% of cases).
- **Norwegian Scabies:** There is orthokeratosis and parakeratosis with many mites in all stages of development. The epidermis shows psoriasiform hyperplasia with mild spongiosis and exocytosis of eosinophils and neutrophils.

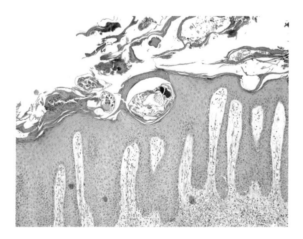

FIGURE 9-29 *Scabies*
Norwegian scabies showing orthokeratosis and parakeratosis with many mites in all stages of development.

Tungiasis

Tungiasis is an infestation by the burrowing pregnant female sand flea Tunga pene-trans. Tungiasis is common in Central America, South America, India, and tropical Africa. Classic areas of involvement include the plantar surface of the foot and the inter-triginous regions of the toes. Infestation is manifested by a white patch with a black dot and eventually the lesions adopt crusted erythematous papules. Secondary infections could result in lymphangitis and septicemia (387, 388).

HISTOLOGY (FIGURE 9-30):
- The tunga can be seen in epidermis or dermis.
- The tunga has a thick cuticle and a band of striated muscle stretching from the head to the abdominal orifice. Also, hollow, ring-shaped elements (tracheal system) and numerous round or oval eggs.
- A mixed inflammatory response composed of lymphocytes, histiocytes, plasma cells, and eosinophils.

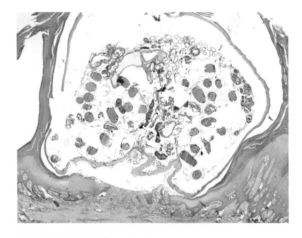

FIGURE 9-30 *Tungiasis*
Tunga showing a thick cuticle and a band of striated muscle stretching from the head to the abdominal orifice.

References

1. Krasteva M. Contact dermatitis. *Int J Dermatol*. 1993;32:547–560.
2. Astner S, Burnett N, Rius-Díaz F, et al. Irritant contact dermatitis induced by a common household irritant: a noninvasive evaluation of ethnic variability in skin response. *J Am Acad Dermatol*. 2006;54:458–465.
3. White CR Jr. Histopathology of exogenous and systemic contact eczema. *Semin Dermatol*. 1990;9:226–229.
4. Hussein MR. Evaluation of Langerhans' cells in normal and eczematous dermatitis skin by CD1a protein immunohistochemistry: preliminary findings. *J Cutan Pathol*. 2008;35:554–558.
5. Hanifin JM. Atopic dermatitis. *J Am Acad Dermatol*. 1982;6:1–13.
6. van Neste D, Douka M, Rahier J, et al. Epidermal changes in atopic dermatitis. *Acta Derm Venereol Suppl (Stockh)*. 1985;114:67–71.
7. Uehara M, Miyauchi H. The morphologic characteristics of dry skin in atopic dermatitis. *Arch Dermatol*. 1984;120:1186–1190.
8. Aoyama H, Tanaka M, Hara M, et al. Nummular eczema: an addition of senile xerosis and unique cutaneous reactivities to environmental aeroallergens. *Dermatology*. 1999;199:135–139.
9. Epstein E. Hand dermatitis: practical management and current concepts. *J Am Acad Dermatol*. 1984;10:395–424.
10. Miller RM, Coger RW. Skin conductance conditioning with dyshidrotic eczema patients. *Br J Dermatol*. 1979;101:435–440.
11. Fox BJ, Odom RB. Papulosquamous diseases: a review. *J Am Acad Dermatol*. 1985;12:597–624.
12. Mathes BM, Douglass MC. Seborrheic dermatitis in patients with acquired immunodeficiency syndrome. *J Am Acad Dermatol*. 1985;13:947–951.
13. Binder RL, Jonelis FJ. Seborrheic dermatitis in neuroleptic-induced parkinsonism. *Arch Dermatol*. 1983;119:473–475.
14. Soeprono FF, Schinella RA, Cockerell CJ, et al. Seborrheic-like dermatitis of acquired immunodeficiency syndrome. A clinicopathologic study. *J Am Acad Dermatol*. 1986;14:242–248.
15. Drago F, Ranieri E, Malaguti F, et al. Human herpesvirus 7 in patients with pityriasis rosea. Electron microscopy investigations and polymerase chain reaction in mononuclear cells, plasma and skin. *Dermatology*. 1997;195:374–378.
16. Parsons JM. Pityriasis rosea update: 1986. *J Am Acad Dermatol*. 1986;15:159–167.
17. Güçlüer H, Gürbüz O, Kotiloglu E. Kaposi-like acroangiodermatitis in an amputee. *Br J Dermatol*. 1999;141:380–381.

18. Landthaler M, Stolz W, Eckert F, et al. Pseudo-Kaposi's sarcoma occurring after placement of arteriovenous shunt. A case report with DNA content analysis. *J Am Acad Dermatol.* 1989;21:499–505.
19. Fry L. Psoriasis. *Br J Dermatol.* 1988;119:445–461.
20. Christophers E. Comorbidities in psoriasis. *Clin Dermatol.* 2007;25:529–534.
21. Christophers E, Kiene P. Guttate and plaque psoriasis. *Dermatol Clin.* 1995;13:751–756.
22. Zelickson BD, Muller SA. Generalized pustular psoriasis. A review of 63 cases. *Arch Dermatol.* 1991;127:1339–1345.
23. Lotti T, Buggiani G, Prignano F. Prurigo nodularis and lichen simplex chronicus. *Dermatol Ther.* 2008;21:42–46.
24. Griffiths WA. Pityriasis rubra pilaris: the problem of its classification. *J Am Acad Dermatol.* 1992;26:140–142.
25. Keat A. Reiter's syndrome and reactive arthritis in perspective. *N Engl J Med.* 1983;309:1606–1615.
26. Leirisalo M, Skylv G, Kousa M, et al. Followup study on patients with Reiter's disease and reactive arthritis, with special reference to HLA-B27. *Arthritis Rheum.* 1982;25:249–259.
27. Hegyi J, Schwartz RA, Hegyi V. Pellagra: dermatitis, dementia, and diarrhea. *Int J Dermatol.* 2004;43:1–5.
28. Karthikeyan K, Thappa DM. Pellagra and skin. *Int J Dermatol.* 2002;41:476–481.
29. Maverakis E, Fung MA, Lynch PJ, et al. Acrodermatitis enteropathica and an overview of zinc metabolism. *J Am Acad Dermatol.* 2007;56:116–124.
30. Evans GW, Johnson PE. Zinc-binding factor in acrodermatitis enteropathica. *Lancet.* 1976;2:1310.
31. Gantcheva ML, Broshtilova VK, Lalova AI. Necrolytic migratory erythema: the outermost marker for glucagonoma syndrome. *Arch Dermatol.* 2007;143:1221–1222.
32. Kahan RS, Perez-Figaredo RA, Neimanis A. Necrolytic migratory erythema. Distinctive dermatosis of the glucagonoma syndrome. *Arch Dermatol.* 1977;113:792–797.
33. Abdallah MA, Ghozzi MY, Monib HA, et al. Necrolytic acral erythema: a cutaneous sign of hepatitis C virus infection. *J Am Acad Dermatol.* 2005;53:247–251.
34. Chuang TY, Stitle L, Brashear R, et al. Hepatitis C virus and lichen planus: a case-control study of 340 patients. *J Am Acad Dermatol.* 1999;41:787–789.
35. Shengyuan L, Songpo Y, Wen W, et al. Hepatitis C virus and lichen planus: a reciprocal association determined by a meta-analysis. *Arch Dermatol.* 2009;145:1040–1047.
36. Singh SK, Saikia UN, Ajith C, et al. Squamous cell carcinoma arising from hypertrophic lichen planus. *J Eur Acad Dermatol Venereol.* 2006;20:745–746.
37. Tan E, Malik R, Quirk CJ. Hypertrophic lichen planus mimicking squamous cell carcinoma. *Australas J Dermatol.* 1998;39:45–47.
38. Miteva L. Bullous lichen planus with nail involvement induced by hepatitis B vaccine in a child. *Int J Dermatol.* 2005;44:142–144.
39. Willsteed E, Bhogal BS, Das AK, et al. Lichen planus pemphigoides: a clinicopathological study of nine cases. *Histopathology.* 1991;19:147–154.
40. Lang PG Jr, Maize JC. Coexisting lichen planus and bullous pemphigoid or lichen planus pemphigoides? *J Am Acad Dermatol.* 1983;9:133–140.
41. Eisen D. The clinical features, malignant potential, and systemic associations of oral lichen planus: a study of 723 patients. *J Am Acad Dermatol.* 2002;46:207–214.
42. Matta M, Kibbi AG, Khattar J, et al. Lichen planopilaris: a clinicopathologic study. *J Am Acad Dermatol.* 1990;22:594–598.
43. Mehregan DA, Van Hale HM, Muller SA. Lichen planopilaris: clinical and pathologic study of forty-five patients. *J Am Acad Dermatol.* 1992;27:935–942.
44. Halevy S, Shai A. Lichenoid drug eruptions. *J Am Acad Dermatol.* 1993;29:249–255.

45. Almeyda J, Levantine A. Drug reactions. XVI. Lichenoid drug eruptions. *Br J Dermatol.* 1971;85:604–607.

46. Morgan MB, Stevens GL, Switlyk S. Benign lichenoid keratosis: a clinical and pathologic reappraisal of 1040 cases. *Am J Dermatopathol.* 2005;27:387–392.

47. Laur WE, Posey RE, Waller JD. Lichen planus-like keratosis. A clinicohistopathologic correlation. *J Am Acad Dermatol.* 1981;4:329–336.

48. Prieto VG, Casal M, McNutt NS. Lichen planus-like keratosis. A clinical and histological reexamination. *Am J Surg Pathol.* 1993;17:259–263.

49. Lapins NA, Willoughby C, Helwig EB. Lichen nitidus. A study of forty-three cases. *Cutis.* 1978;21:634–637.

50. Zhang Y, McNutt NS. Lichen striatus. Histological, immunohistochemical, and ultrastructural study of 37 cases. *J Cutan Pathol.* 2001;28:65–71.

51. Kennedy D, Rogers M. Lichen striatus. *Pediatr Dermatol.* 1996;13:95–99.

52. Hauber K, Rose C, Bröcker EB, et al. Lichen striatus: clinical features and follow-up in 12 patients. *Eur J Dermatol.* 2000;10:536–539.

53. Chan I, Oyama N, Neill SM, et al. Characterization of IgG autoantibodies to extracellular matrix protein 1 in lichen sclerosus. *Clin Exp Dermatol.* 2004;29:499–504.

54. Ridley CM. Lichen sclerosus et atrophicus. *Semin Dermatol.* 1989;8:54–63.

55. Slater DN, Wagner BE. Early vulvar lichen sclerosus: a histopathological challenge. *Histopathology.* 2007;50:388–389; author reply 389–391.

56. Fernandes NF, Rozdeba PJ, Schwartz RA, et al. Pityriasis lichenoides et varioliformis acuta: a disease spectrum. *Int J Dermatol.* 2010;49:257–261.

57. Bowers S, Warshaw EM. Pityriasis lichenoides and its subtypes. *J Am Acad Dermatol.* 2006;55:557–572; quiz 573–576.

58. Magro CM, Crowson AN, Morrison C, et al. Pityriasis lichenoides chronica: stratification by molecular and phenotypic profile. *Hum Pathol.* 2007;38:479–490.

59. Magro C, Crowson AN, Kovatich A, et al. Pityriasis lichenoides: a clonal T-cell lymphoproliferative disorder. *Hum Pathol.* 2002;33:788–795.

60. Tonnesen MG, Soter NA. Erythema multiforme. *J Am Acad Dermatol.* 1979;1:357–364.

61. Huff JC, Weston WL, Tonnesen MG. Erythema multiforme: a critical review of characteristics, diagnostic criteria, and causes. *J Am Acad Dermatol.* 1983;8:763–775.

62. Howland WW, Golitz LE, Weston WL, et al. Erythema multiforme: clinical, histopathologic, and immunologic study. *J Am Acad Dermatol.* 1984;10:438–446.

63. Justiniano H, Berlingeri-Ramos AC, Sánchez JL. Pattern analysis of drug-induced skin diseases. *Am J Dermatopathol.* 2008;30:352–369.

64. Wintroub BU, Stern R. Cutaneous drug reactions: pathogenesis and clinical classification. *J Am Acad Dermatol.* 1985;13:167–179.

65. Clark WH, Reed RJ, Mihm MC. Lupus erythematosus. Histopathology of cutaneous lesions. *Hum Pathol.* 1973;4:157–163.

66. Gilliam JN, Sontheimer RD. Distinctive cutaneous subsets in the spectrum of lupus erythematosus. *J Am Acad Dermatol.* 1981;4:471–475.

67. Chieregato C, Barba A, Zini A, et al. Discoid lupus erythematosus: clinical and pathological study of 24 patients. *J Eur Acad Dermatol Venereol.* 2004;18:113.

68. Prystowsky SD, Gilliam JN. Discoid lupus erythematosus as part of a larger disease spectrum. Correlation of clinical features with laboratory findings in lupus erythematosus. *Arch Dermatol.* 1975;111:1448–1452.

69. Vieira V, Del Pozo J, Yebra-Pimentel MT, et al. Lupus erythematosus tumidus: a series of 26 cases. *Int J Dermatol.* 2006;45:512–517.

70. Dekle CL, Mannes KD, Davis LS, et al. Lupus tumidus. *J Am Acad Dermatol.* 1999;41:250–253.

71. Harper JI. Subacute cutaneous lupus erythematosus (SCLE): a distinct subset of LE. *Clin Exp Dermatol*. 1982;7:209–212.
72. Black DR, Hornung CA, Schneider PD, et al. Frequency and severity of systemic disease in patients with subacute cutaneous lupus erythematosus. *Arch Dermatol*. 2002;138: 1175–1178.
73. Callen JP, Hughes AP, Kulp-Shorten C. Subacute cutaneous lupus erythematosus induced or exacerbated by terbinafine: a report of 5 cases. *Arch Dermatol*. 2001;137:1196–1198.
74. Goodfield M. Measuring the activity of disease in cutaneous lupus erythematosus. *Br J Dermatol*. 2000;142:399–400.
75. Lee LA, Weston WL. Neonatal lupus erythematosus. *Semin Dermatol*. 1988;7:66–72.
76. Hogan PA. Neonatal lupus erythematosus. *Australas J Dermatol*. 1995;36:39–40.
77. Kovacs SO, Kovacs SC. Dermatomyositis. *J Am Acad Dermatol*. 1998;39:899–920; quiz 921–922.
78. Callen JP. Dermatomyositis. *Lancet*. 2000;355:53–57.
79. Janis JF, Winkelmann RK. Histopathology of the skin in dermatomyositis. A histopathologic study of 55 cases. *Arch Dermatol*. 1968;97:640–650.
80. Korkij W, Soltani K. Fixed drug eruption. A brief review. *Arch Dermatol*. 1984;120:520–524.
81. Shukla SR. Drugs causing fixed drug eruptions. *Dermatologica*. 1981;163:160–163.
82. Hood AF, Soter NA, Rappeport J, et al. Graft-versus-host reaction. Cutaneous manifestations following bone marrow transplantation. *Arch Dermatol*. 1977;113:1087–1091.
83. Johnson ML, Farmer ER. Graft-versus-host reactions in dermatology. *J Am Acad Dermatol*. 1998;38:369–392; quiz 393–396.
84. Hymes SR, Farmer ER, Lewis PG, et al. Cutaneous graft-versus-host reaction: prognostic features seen by light microscopy. *J Am Acad Dermatol*. 1985;12:468–474.
85. Bystryn JC, Moore MM. Cutaneous pemphigus vulgaris: what causes it? *J Am Acad Dermatol*. 2006;55:175–176; author reply 176–177.
86. Ahmed AR. Clinical features of pemphigus. *Clin Dermatol*. 1983;1:13–21.
87. Plott RT, Amagai M, Udey MC, et al. Pemphigus vulgaris antigen lacks biochemical properties characteristic of classical cadherins. *J Invest Dermatol*. 1994;103:168–172.
88. Iwatsuki K, Takigawa M, Imaizumi S, et al. In vivo binding site of pemphigus vulgaris antibodies and their fate during acantholysis. *J Am Acad Dermatol*. 1989;20:578–582.
89. Shapiro M, Jimenez S, Werth VP. Pemphigus vulgaris induced by D-penicillamine therapy in a patient with systemic sclerosis. *J Am Acad Dermatol*. 2000;42:297–299.
90. Judd KP, Lever WF. Correlation of antibodies in skin and serum with disease severity in pemphigus. *Arch Dermatol*. 1979;115:428–432.
91. Koulu L, Stanley JR. Clinical, histologic, and immunopathologic comparison of pemphigus vulgaris and pemphigus foliaceus. *Semin Dermatol*. 1988;7:82–90.
92. Diaz LA, Sampaio SA, Rivitti EA, et al. Endemic pemphigus foliaceus (fogo selvagem). I. Clinical features and immunopathology. *J Am Acad Dermatol*. 1989;20:657–669.
93. Rubinstein N, Stanley JR. Pemphigus foliaceus antibodies and a monoclonal antibody to desmoglein I demonstrate stratified squamous epithelial-specific epitopes of desmosomes. *Am J Dermatopathol*. 1987;9:510–514.
94. Camisa C, Helm TN. Paraneoplastic pemphigus is a distinct neoplasia-induced autoimmune disease. *Arch Dermatol*. 1993;129:883–886.
95. Wade MS, Black MM. Paraneoplastic pemphigus: a brief update. *Australas J Dermatol*. 2005;46:1–8; quiz 9–10.
96. Ahmed AR, Blose DA. Pemphigus vegetans. Neumann type and Hallopeau type. *Int J Dermatol*. 1984;23:135–141.
97. Niimi Y, Kawana S, Kusunoki T. IgA pemphigus: a case report and its characteristic clinical features compared with subcorneal pustular dermatosis. *J Am Acad Dermatol*. 2000;43:546–549.

98. Yasuda H, Kobayashi H, Hashimoto T, et al. Subcorneal pustular dermatosis type of IgA pemphigus: demonstration of autoantibodies to desmocollin-1 and clinical review. *Br J Dermatol.* 2000;143:144–148.

99. Michel B. "Familial benign chronic pemphigus" by Hailey and Hailey, April 1939. Commentary: Hailey-Hailey disease, familial benign chronic pemphigus. *Arch Dermatol.* 1982;118:774–783.

100. Chave TA, Milligan A. Acute generalized Hailey-Hailey disease. *Clin Exp Dermatol.* 2002;27:290–292.

101. Sudbrak R, Brown J, Dobson-Stone C, et al. Hailey-Hailey disease is caused by mutations in ATP2C1 encoding a novel Ca(2+) pump. *Hum Mol Genet.* 2000;9:1131–1140.

102. Burge SM, Wilkinson JD. Darier-White disease: a review of the clinical features in 163 patients. *J Am Acad Dermatol.* 1992;27:40–50.

103. Burge S. Darier's disease—the clinical features and pathogenesis. *Clin Exp Dermatol.* 1994;19:193–205.

104. Sheridan AT, Hollowood K, Sakuntabhai A, et al. Expression of sarco/endo-plasmic reticulum Ca2+-ATPase type 2 isoforms (SERCA2) in normal human skin and mucosa, and Darier's disease skin. *Br J Dermatol.* 2002;147:670–674.

105. Grover RW. Transient acantholytic dermatosis. *Arch Dermatol.* 1970;101:426–434.

106. Chalet M, Grover R, Ackerman AB. Transient acantholytic dermatosis: a reevaluation. *Arch Dermatol.* 1977;113:431–435.

107. Braun-Falco M, Volgger W, Borelli S, et al. Galli-Galli disease: an unrecognized entity or an acantholytic variant of Dowling-Degos disease? *J Am Acad Dermatol.* 2001;45:760–763.

108. Bundino S, Zina AM, Ubertalli S. Infantile acropustulosis. *Dermatologica.* 1982;165:615–619.

109. Newton JA, Salisbury J, Marsden A, et al. Acropustulosis of infancy. *Br J Dermatol.* 1986;115:735–739.

110. Ramamurthy RS, Reveri M, Esterly NB, et al. Transient neonatal pustular melanosis. *J Pediatr.* 1976;88:831–835.

111. Barr RJ, Globerman LM, Werber FA. Transient neonatal pustular melanosis. *Int J Dermatol.* 1979;18:636–638.

112. Freeman RG, Spiller R, Knox JM. Histopathology of erythema toxicum neonatorum. *Arch Dermatol.* 1960;82:586–589.

113. Schachner L, Press S. Vesicular, bullous and pustular disorders in infancy and childhood. *Pediatr Clin North Am.* 1983;30:609–629.

114. Vaillant L, Bernard P, Joly P, et al. Evaluation of clinical criteria for diagnosis of bullous pemphigoid. French Bullous Study Group. *Arch Dermatol.* 1998;134:1075–1080.

115. Wong SN, Chua SH. Spectrum of subepidermal immunobullous disorders seen at the National Skin Centre, Singapore: a 2-year review. *Br J Dermatol.* 2002;147:476–480.

116. Korman N. Bullous pemphigoid. *J Am Acad Dermatol.* 1987;16:907–924.

117. Cook AL, Hanahoe TH, Mallett RB, et al. Recognition of two distinct major antigens by bullous pemphigoid sera. *Br J Dermatol.* 1990;122:435–444.

118. Nishioka K, Hashimoto K, Katayama I, et al. Eosinophilic spongiosis in bullous pemphigoid. *Arch Dermatol.* 1984;120:1166–1168.

119. Bernard P, Prost C, Durepaire N, et al. The major cicatricial pemphigoid antigen is a 180-kD protein that shows immunologic cross-reactivities with the bullous pemphigoid antigen. *J Invest Dermatol.* 1992;99:174–179.

120. Mimouni D, Anhalt GJ, Lazarova Z, et al. Paraneoplastic pemphigus in children and adolescents. *Br J Dermatol.* 2002;147:725–732.

121. Fleming TE, Korman NJ. Cicatricial pemphigoid. *J Am Acad Dermatol.* 2000;43:571–591; quiz 591–594.

122. Holmes RC, Black MM. The specific dermatoses of pregnancy. *J Am Acad Dermatol.* 1983;8:405–412.

123. Shornick JK. Herpes gestationis. *J Am Acad Dermatol*. 1987;17:539–556.
124. Chimanovitch I, Schmidt E, Messer G, et al. IgG1 and IgG3 are the major immunoglobulin subclasses targeting epitopes within the NC16A domain of BP180 in pemphigoid gestationis. *J Invest Dermatol*. 1999;113:140–142.
125. Faure M. Dermatitis herpetiformis. *Semin Dermatol*. 1988;7:123–129.
126. Thiers BH. Dermatitis herpetiformis. *J Am Acad Dermatol*. 1981;5:114–117.
127. Oxentenko AS, Murray JA. Celiac disease and dermatitis herpetiformis: the spectrum of gluten-sensitive enteropathy. *Int J Dermatol*. 2003;42:585–587.
128. Hall RP. The pathogenesis of dermatitis herpetiformis: recent advances. *J Am Acad Dermatol*. 1987;16:1129–1144.
129. Wojnarowska F, Marsden RA, Bhogal B, et al. Chronic bullous disease of childhood, childhood cicatricial pemphigoid, and linear IgA disease of adults. A comparative study demonstrating clinical and immunopathologic overlap. *J Am Acad Dermatol*. 1988;19:792–805.
130. Leonard JN, Haffenden GP, Ring NP, et al. Linear IgA disease in adults. *Br J Dermatol*. 1982;107:301–316.
131. Wojnarowska F, Collier PM, Allen J, et al. The localization of the target antigens and antibodies in linear IgA disease is heterogeneous, and dependent on the methods used. *Br J Dermatol*. 1995;132:750–757.
132. Marinkovich MP, Taylor TB, Keene DR, et al. LAD-1, the linear IgA bullous dermatosis autoantigen, is a novel 120-kDa anchoring filament protein synthesized by epidermal cells. *J Invest Dermatol*. 1996;106:734–738.
133. Fujimoto W, Hamada T, Yamada J, et al. Bullous systemic lupus erythematosus as an Initial manifestation of SLE. *J Dermatol*. 2005;32:1021–1027.
134. Chan LS, Lapiere JC, Chen M, et al. Bullous systemic lupus erythematosus with autoantibodies recognizing multiple skin basement membrane components, bullous pemphigoid antigen 1, laminin-5, laminin-6, and type VII collagen. *Arch Dermatol*. 1999;135:569–573.
135. Bleasel NR, Varigos GA. Porphyria cutanea tarda. *Australas J Dermatol*. 2000;41:197–206; quiz 207–208.
136. Méndez M, Rossetti MV, Del CBAM, et al. The role of inherited and acquired factors in the development of porphyria cutanea tarda in the Argentinean population. *J Am Acad Dermatol*. 2005;52:417–424.
137. O'Reilly K, Snape J, Moore MR. Porphyria cutanea tarda resulting from primary hepatocellular carcinoma. *Clin Exp Dermatol*. 1988;13:44–48.
138. Pearson RW. Clinicopathologic types of epidermolysis bullosa and their nondermatological complications. *Arch Dermatol*. 1988;124:718–725.
139. Haber RM, Hanna W, Ramsay CA, et al. Hereditary epidermolysis bullosa. *J Am Acad Dermatol*. 1985;13:252–278.
140. Sanchez G, Seltzer JL, Eisen AZ, et al. Generalized dominant epidermolysis bullosa simplex: decreased activity of a gelatinolytic protease in cultured fibroblasts as a phenotypic marker. *J Invest Dermatol*. 1983;81:576–579.
141. Gil SG, Brown TA, Ryan MC, et al. Junctional epidermolysis bullosis: defects in expression of epiligrin/nicein/kalinin and integrin beta 4 that inhibit hemidesmosome formation. *J Invest Dermatol*. 1994;103:31S–38S.
142. Horn HM, Tidman MJ. The clinical spectrum of dystrophic epidermolysis bullosa. *Br J Dermatol*. 2002;146:267–274.
143. Prieto VG, McNutt NS. Immunohistochemical detection of keratin with the monoclonal antibody MNF116 is useful in the diagnosis of epidermolysis bullosa simplex. *J Cutan Pathol*. 1994;21:118–122.
144. Gammon WR. Epidermolysis bullosa acquisita. *Semin Dermatol*. 1988;7:218–224.
145. Mihai S, Sitaru C. Immunopathology and molecular diagnosis of autoimmune bullous diseases. *J Cell Mol Med*. 2007;11:462–481.

146. Gammon WR, Briggaman RA. Functional heterogeneity of immune complexes in epidermolysis bullosa acquisita. *J Invest Dermatol*. 1987;89:478–483.

147a. Prieto VG, Sadick NS, McNutt NS. Quantitative immunohistochemical differences in Langerhans cells in dermatitis due to internal versus external antigen sources. *J Cutan Pathol* 25(6):301-10, 7/1998).

147b. Synkowski D, Dore N, Provost TT. Urticaria and Urticaria-like lesions. *Clin Rheum Dis*. 1982;8:383–395.

148. Sánchez JL, Benmamán O. Clinicopathological correlation in chronic urticaria. *Am J Dermatopathol*. 1992;14:220–223.

149. Kiszewski AE, Durán-Mckinster C, Orozco-Covarrubias L, et al. Cutaneous mastocytosis in children: a clinical analysis of 71 cases. *J Eur Acad Dermatol Venereol*. 2004;18:285–290.

150. Azaña JM, Torrelo A, Mediero IG, et al. Urticaria pigmentosa: a review of 67 pediatric cases. *Pediatr Dermatol*. 1994;11:102–106.

151. Gibbs NF, Friedlander SF, Harpster EF. Telangiectasia macularis eruptiva perstans. *Pediatr Dermatol*. 2000;17:194–197.

152. Lacz NL, Vafaie J, Kihiczak NI, et al. Postinflammatory hyperpigmentation: a common but troubling condition. *Int J Dermatol*. 2004;43:362–365.

153. Rudolph CM, Al-Fares S, Vaughan-Jones SA, et al. Polymorphic eruption of pregnancy: clinicopathology and potential trigger factors in 181 patients. *Br J Dermatol*. 2006;154:54–60.

154. Krinsky WL. Dermatoses associated with the bites of mites and ticks (Arthropoda: Acari). *Int J Dermatol*. 1983;22:75–91.

155. Sams HH, Dunnick CA, Smith ML, et al. Necrotic arachnidism. *J Am Acad Dermatol*. 2001;44:561–573; quiz 573–576.

156. Boonstra HE, van Weelden H, Toonstra J, et al. Polymorphous light eruption: a clinical, photobiologic, and follow-up study of 110 patients. *J Am Acad Dermatol*. 2000;42:199–207.

157. Kim KJ, Chang SE, Choi JH, et al. Clinicopathologic analysis of 66 cases of erythema annulare centrifugum. *J Dermatol*. 2002;29:61–67.

158. Eubanks LE, McBurney E, Reed R. Erythema gyratum repens. *Am J Med Sci*. 2001;321:302–305.

159. Sweet RD. An acute febrile neutrophilic dermatosis. *Br J Dermatol*. 1964;76:349–356.

160. Weenig RH, Bruce AJ, McEvoy MT, et al. Neutrophilic dermatosis of the hands: four new cases and review of the literature. *Int J Dermatol*. 2004;43:95–102.

161. Jordaan HF. Acute febrile neutrophilic dermatosis. A histopathological study of 37 patients and a review of the literature. *Am J Dermatopathol*. 1989;11:99–111.

162. Jorizzo JL, Solomon AR, Zanolli MD, et al. Neutrophilic vascular reactions. *J Am Acad Dermatol*. 1988;19:983–1005.

163. Callen JP, Jackson JM. Pyoderma gangrenosum: an update. *Rheum Dis Clin North Am*. 2007;33:787–802, vi.

164. Wood C, Miller AC, Jacobs A, et al. Eosinophilic infiltration with flame figures. A distinctive tissue reaction seen in Wells' syndrome and other diseases. *Am J Dermatopathol*. 1986;8:186–193.

165. Modlin RL, Vaccaro SA, Gottlieb B, et al. Granuloma annulare. Identification of cells in the cutaneous infiltrate by immunoperoxidase techniques. *Arch Pathol Lab Med*. 1984;108:379–382.

166. Zanolli MD, Powell BL, McCalmont T, et al. Granuloma annulare and disseminated herpes zoster. *Int J Dermatol*. 1992;31:55–57.

167. Mutasim DF, Bridges AG. Patch granuloma annulare: clinicopathologic study of 6 patients. *J Am Acad Dermatol*. 2000;42:417–421.

168. O'Brien JP, Regan W. Actinically degenerate elastic tissue is the likely antigenic basis of actinic granuloma of the skin and of temporal arteritis. *J Am Acad Dermatol*. 1999;40:214–222.

169. Johnson WC. Necrobiotic granulomas. *J Cutan Pathol.* 1985;12:289–299.
170. Muller SA, Winkelmann RK. Necrobiosis lipoidica diabeticorum histopathologic study of 98 cases. *Arch Dermatol.* 1966;94:1–10.
171. Mehregan DA, Winkelmann RK. Necrobiotic xanthogranuloma. *Arch Dermatol.* 1992;128:94–100.
172. Patterson JW. Rheumatoid nodule and subcutaneous granuloma annulare. A comparative histologic study. *Am J Dermatopathol.* 1988;10:1–8.
173. Hanno R, Callen JP. Sarcoidosis: a disorder with prominent cutaneous features and their interrelationship with systemic disease. *Med Clin North Am.* 1980;64:847–866.
174. Walsh NM, Hanly JG, Tremaine R, et al. Cutaneous sarcoidosis and foreign bodies. *Am J Dermatopathol.* 1993;15:203–207.
175. Greene RM, Rogers RS III. Melkersson-Rosenthal syndrome: a review of 36 patients. *J Am Acad Dermatol.* 1989;21:1263–1270.
176. Zelger B, Cerio R, Soyer HP, et al. Reticulohistiocytoma and multicentric reticulohistiocytosis. Histopathologic and immunophenotypic distinct entities. *Am J Dermatopathol.* 1994;16:577–584.
177. Oliver GF, Umbert I, Winkelmann RK, et al. Reticulohistiocytoma cutis—review of 15 cases and an association with systemic vasculitis in two cases. *Clin Exp Dermatol.* 1990;15:1–6.
178. Sangüeza OP, Salmon JK, White CR Jr, et al. Juvenile xanthogranuloma: a clinical, histopathologic and immunohistochemical study. *J Cutan Pathol.* 1995;22:327–335.
179. Zelger B, Cerio R, Orchard G, et al. Juvenile and adult xanthogranuloma. A histological and immunohistochemical comparison. *Am J Surg Pathol.* 1994;18:126–135.
180. Gianotti R, Alessi E, Caputo R. Benign cephalic histiocytosis: a distinct entity or a part of a wide spectrum of histiocytic proliferative disorders of children? A histopathological study. *Am J Dermatopathol.* 1993;15:315–319.
181. Chu P, Connolly MK, LeBoit PE. The histopathologic spectrum of palisaded neutrophilic and granulomatous dermatitis in patients with collagen vascular disease. *Arch Dermatol.* 1994;130:1278–1283.
182. Magro CM, Crowson AN, Regauer S. Granuloma annulare and necrobiosis lipoidica tissue reactions as a manifestation of systemic disease. *Hum Pathol.* 1996;27:50–56.
183. Jennette JC, Falk RJ, Andrassy K, et al. Nomenclature of systemic vasculitides. Proposal of an international consensus conference. *Arthritis Rheum.* 1994;37:187–192.
184. LeBoit PE. Dust to dust. *Am J Dermatopathol.* 2005;27:277–278.
185. Pinkus H. [Facial granuloma]. *Dermatologica.* 1952;105:85–99.
186. LeBoit PE, Yen TS, Wintroub B. The evolution of lesions in erythema elevatum diutinum. *Am J Dermatopathol.* 1986;8:392–402.
187. Requena L, Sánchez Yus E, Martín L, et al. Erythema elevatum diutinum in a patient with acquired immunodeficiency syndrome. Another clinical simulator of Kaposi's sarcoma. *Arch Dermatol.* 1991;127:1819–1822.
188. Díaz-Pérez JL, De Lagrán ZM, Diaz-Ramón JL, et al. Cutaneous polyarteritis nodosa. *Semin Cutan Med Surg.* 2007;26:77–86.
189. Davis MD, Daoud MS, McEvoy MT, et al. Cutaneous manifestations of Churg-Strauss syndrome: a clinicopathologic correlation. *J Am Acad Dermatol.* 1997;37:199–203.
190. Chen KR, Sakamoto M, Ikemoto K, et al. Granulomatous arteritis in cutaneous lesions of Churg-Strauss syndrome. *J Cutan Pathol.* 2007;34:330–337.
191. Godman GC, Churg J. Wegener's granulomatosis: pathology and review of the literature. *AMA Arch Pathol.* 1954;58:533–553.
192. Comfere NI, Macaron NC, Gibson LE. Cutaneous manifestations of Wegener's granulomatosis: a clinicopathologic study of 17 patients and correlation to antineutrophil cytoplasmic antibody status. *J Cutan Pathol.* 2007;34:739–747.

193. Barksdale SK, Hallahan CW, Kerr GS, et al. Cutaneous pathology in Wegener's granulomatosis. A clinicopathologic study of 75 biopsies in 46 patients. *Am J Surg Pathol.* 1995;19:161–172.
194. Randall SJ, Kierland RR, Montgomery H. Pigmented purpuric eruptions. *AMA Arch Derm Syphilol.* 1951;64:177–191.
195. Barnhill RL, Braverman IM. Progression of pigmented purpura-like eruptions to mycosis fungoides: report of three cases. *J Am Acad Dermatol.* 1988;19:25–31.
196. Sansonno D, Dammacco F. Hepatitis C virus, cryoglobulinaemia, and vasculitis: immune complex relations. *Lancet Infect Dis.* 2005;5:227–236.
197. Cohen SJ, Pittelkow MR, Su WP. Cutaneous manifestations of cryoglobulinemia: clinical and histopathologic study of seventy-two patients. *J Am Acad Dermatol.* 1991;25:21–27.
198. Harvell JD, Williford PL, White WL. Benign cutaneous Degos' disease: a case report with emphasis on histopathology as papules chronologically evolve. *Am J Dermatopathol.* 2001;23:116–123.
199. Stiefler RE, Bergfeld WF. Atrophie blanche. *Int J Dermatol.* 1982;21:1–7.
200. Fischer AH, Morris DJ. Pathogenesis of calciphylaxis: study of three cases with literature review. *Hum Pathol.* 1995;26:1055–1064.
201. Ferreres JR, Marcoval J, Bordas X, et al. Calciphylaxis associated with alcoholic cirrhosis. *J Eur Acad Dermatol Venereol.* 2006;20:599–601.
202. Hampl JS, Taylor CA, Johnston CS. Vitamin C deficiency and depletion in the United States: the Third National Health and Nutrition Examination Survey, 1988 to 1994. *Am J Public Health.* 2004;94:870–875.
203. Ghorbani AJ, Eichler C. Scurvy. *J Am Acad Dermatol.* 1994;30:881–883.
204. Uitto J, Santa Cruz DJ, Bauer EA, et al. Morphea and lichen sclerosus et atrophicus. Clinical and histopathologic studies in patients with combined features. *J Am Acad Dermatol.* 1980;3:271–279.
205. Su WP, Person JR. Morphea profunda. A new concept and a histopathologic study of 23 cases. *Am J Dermatopathol.* 1981;3:251–260.
206. LeRoy EC, Black C, Fleischmajer R, et al. Scleroderma (systemic sclerosis): classification, subsets and pathogenesis. *J Rheumatol.* 1988;15:202–205.
207. Krieg T, Meurer M. Systemic scleroderma. Clinical and pathophysiologic aspects. *J Am Acad Dermatol.* 1988;18:457–481.
208. Shabana WM, Cohan RH, Ellis JH, et al. Nephrogenic systemic fibrosis: a report of 29 cases. *AJR Am J Roentgenol.* 2008;190:736–741.
209. Deng A, Martin DB, Spillane A, et al. Nephrogenic systemic fibrosis with a spectrum of clinical and histopathological presentation: a disorder of aberrant dermal remodeling. *J Cutan Pathol.* 2010;37:204–210.
210. LeBoit PE. Subacute radiation dermatitis: a histologic imitator of acute cutaneous graft-versus-host disease. *J Am Acad Dermatol.* 1989;20:236–241.
211. Pope FM. Historical evidence for the genetic heterogeneity of pseudoxanthoma elasticum. *Br J Dermatol.* 1975;92:493–509.
212. Bergen AA, Plomp AS, Schuurman EJ, et al. Mutations in ABCC6 cause pseudoxanthoma elasticum. *Nat Genet.* 2000;25:228–231.
213. Chanda JJ, Callen JP, Taylor WB. Diffuse fasciitis with eosinophilia. *Arch Dermatol.* 1978;114:1522–1524.
214. Falanga V, Medsger TA Jr. Frequency, levels, and significance of blood eosinophilia in systemic sclerosis, localized scleroderma, and eosinophilic fasciitis. *J Am Acad Dermatol.* 1987;17:648–656.
215. Uitto J, Santa-Cruz DJ, Eisen AZ. Familial cutaneous collagenoma: genetic studies on a family. *Br J Dermatol.* 1979;101:185–195.

216. Pierard GE, Lapiere CM. Nevi of connective tissue. A reappraisal of their classification. *Am J Dermatopathol*. 1985;7:325–333.
217. Staughton RC. Focal dermal hypoplasia. *Proc R Soc Med*. 1976;69:232–233.
218. Goltz RW, Henderson RR, Hitch JM, et al. Focal dermal hypoplasia syndrome. A review of the literature and report of two cases. *Arch Dermatol*. 1970;101:1–11.
219. Hood AF, Hardegen GL, Zarate AR, et al. Kyrle's disease in patients with chronic renal failure. *Arch Dermatol*. 1982;118:85–88.
220. Rapini RP, Herbert AA, Drucker CR. Acquired perforating dermatosis. Evidence for combined transepidermal elimination of both collagen and elastic fibers. *Arch Dermatol*. 1989;125:1074–1078.
221. Mehregan AH. Elastosis perforans serpiginosa: a review of the literature and report of 11 cases. *Arch Dermatol*. 1968;97:381–393.
222. Mehregan AH, Coskey RJ. Perforating folliculitis. *Arch Dermatol*. 1968;97:394–399.
223. Patterson JW. The perforating disorders. *J Am Acad Dermatol*. 1984;10:561–581.
224. Faver IR, Daoud MS, Su WP. Acquired reactive perforating collagenosis. Report of six cases and review of the literature. *J Am Acad Dermatol*. 1994;30:575–580.
225. Requena L, Yus ES. Panniculitis. Part I. Mostly septal panniculitis. *J Am Acad Dermatol*. 2001;45:163–183; quiz 184–186.
226. Winkelmann RK, Förström L. New observations in the histopathology of erythema nodosum. *J Invest Dermatol*. 1975;65:441–446.
227. Sanchez Yus E, Sanz Vico MD, de Diego V. Miescher's radial granuloma. A characteristic marker of erythema nodosum. *Am J Dermatopathol*. 1989;11:434–442.
228. Poelman SM, Nguyen K. Pancreatic panniculitis associated with acinar cell pancreatic carcinoma. *J Cutan Med Surg*. 2008;12:38–42.
229. Black MM. Panniculitis. *J Cutan Pathol*. 1985;12:366–380.
230. Smith KC, Pittelkow MR, Su WP. Panniculitis associated with severe alpha 1-antitrypsin deficiency. Treatment and review of the literature. *Arch Dermatol*. 1987;123:1655–1661.
231. Su WP, Smith KC, Pittelkow MR, et al. Alpha 1-antitrypsin deficiency panniculitis: a histopathologic and immunopathologic study of four cases. *Am J Dermatopathol*. 1987;9:483–490.
232. Requena L, Sánchez Yus E. Panniculitis. Part II. Mostly lobular panniculitis. *J Am Acad Dermatol*. 2001;45:325–361; quiz 362–364.
233. Rademaker M, Lowe DG, Munro DD. Erythema induratum (Bazin's disease). *J Am Acad Dermatol*. 1989;21:740–745.
234. Burden AD, Krafchik BR. Subcutaneous fat necrosis of the newborn: a review of 11 cases. *Pediatr Dermatol*. 1999;16:384–387.
235. Tuffanelli DL. Lupus erythematosus panniculitis (profundus). *Arch Dermatol*. 1971;103:231–242.
236. Sánchez NP, Peters MS, Winkelmann RK. The histopathology of lupus erythematosus panniculitis. *J Am Acad Dermatol*. 1981;5:673–680.
237. Grossberg E, Scherschun L, Fivenson DP. Lupus profundus: not a benign disease. *Lupus*. 2001;10:514–516.
238. Kirsner RS, Pardes JB, Eaglstein WH, et al. The clinical spectrum of lipodermatosclerosis. *J Am Acad Dermatol*. 1993;28:623–627.
239. Bruce AJ, Bennett DD, Lohse CM, et al. Lipodermatosclerosis: review of cases evaluated at Mayo Clinic. *J Am Acad Dermatol*. 2002;46:187–192.
240. Rongioletti F, Rebora A. Cutaneous mucinoses: microscopic criteria for diagnosis. *Am J Dermatopathol*. 2001;23:257–267.
241. Rongioletti F, Rebora A. Updated classification of papular mucinosis, lichen myxedematosus, and scleromyxedema. *J Am Acad Dermatol*. 2001;44:273–281.
242. Beers WH, Ince A, Moore TL. Scleredema adultorum of Buschke: a case report and review of the literature. *Semin Arthritis Rheum*. 2006;35:355–359.

243. Tominaga A, Tajima S, Ishibashi A, et al. Reticular erythematous mucinosis syndrome with an infiltration of factor XIIIa+ and hyaluronan synthase 2+ dermal dendrocytes. *Br J Dermatol*. 2001;145:141–145.

244. Sonnex TS. Digital myxoid cysts: a review. *Cutis*. 1986;37:89–94.

245. Wilk M, Schmoeckel C. Cutaneous focal mucinosis—a histopathological and immunohistochemical analysis of 11 cases. *J Cutan Pathol*. 1994;21:446–452.

246. Wong CK. Mucocutaneous manifestations in systemic amyloidosis. *Clin Dermatol*. 1990;8:7–12.

247. Breathnach SM. Amyloid and amyloidosis. *J Am Acad Dermatol*. 1988;18:1–16.

248. Moon AO, Calamia KT, Walsh JS. Nodular amyloidosis: review and long-term follow-up of 16 cases. *Arch Dermatol*. 2003;139:1157–1159.

249. Black MM, Jones EW. Macular amyloidosis. A study of 21 cases with special reference to the role of the epidermis in its histogenesis. *Br J Dermatol*. 1971;84:199–209.

250. Weyers W, Weyers I, Bonczkowitz M, et al. Lichen amyloidosus: a consequence of scratching. *J Am Acad Dermatol*. 1997;37:923–928.

251. Touart DM, Sau P. Cutaneous deposition diseases. Part II. *J Am Acad Dermatol*. 1998; 39:527–544; quiz 545–546.

252. Desai AM, Pielop JA, Smith-Zagone MJ, et al. Colloid milium: a histopathologic mimicker of nodular amyloidosis. *Arch Dermatol*. 2006;142:784–785.

253. Hamada T, McLean WH, Ramsay M, et al. Lipoid proteinosis maps to 1q21 and is caused by mutations in the extracellular matrix protein 1 gene (ECM1). *Hum Mol Genet*. 2002;11:833–840.

254. Hamada T. Lipoid proteinosis. *Clin Exp Dermatol*. 2002;27:624–629.

255. Williford PM, White WL, Jorizzo JL, et al. The spectrum of normolipemic plane xanthoma. *Am J Dermatopathol*. 1993;15:572–575.

256. Walsh NM, Murray S, D'Intino Y. Eruptive xanthomata with urate-like crystals. *J Cutan Pathol*. 1994;21:350–355.

257. Smith KJ, Skelton HG, Angritt P. Changes of verruciform xanthoma in an HIV-1+ patient with diffuse psoriasiform skin disease. *Am J Dermatopathol*. 1995;17:185–188.

258. Lesesky EB, Pelle MT, O'Grady TC. Diffuse nodules in a woman with renal failure: chronic tophaceous gout. *Arch Dermatol*. 2007;143:1201–1206.

259. Lawrence N, Bligard CA, Reed R, et al. Exogenous ochronosis in the United States. *J Am Acad Dermatol*. 1988;18:1207–1211.

260. Prose PH. An electron microscopic study of human generalized argyria. *Am J Pathol*. 1963;42:293–299.

261. Berlin AL, Paller AS, Chan LS. Incontinentia pigmenti: a review and update on the molecular basis of pathophysiology. *J Am Acad Dermatol*. 2002;47:169–187; quiz 188–190.

262. Ardelean D, Pope E. Incontinentia pigmenti in boys: a series and review of the literature. *Pediatr Dermatol*. 2006;23:523–527.

263. Ito M, Fujiwara H, Maruyama T, et al. Morphogenesis of the cornoid lamella: histochemical, immunohistochemical, and ultrastructural study of porokeratosis. *J Cutan Pathol*. 1991;18:247–256.

264. Schamroth JM, Zlotogorski A, Gilead L. Porokeratosis of Mibelli. Overview and review of the literature. *Acta Derm Venereol*. 1997;77:207–213.

265. DiGiovanna JJ, Robinson-Bostom L. Ichthyosis: etiology, diagnosis, and management. *Am J Clin Dermatol*. 2003;4:81–95.

266. Mevorah B, Krayenbuhl A, Bovey EH, et al. Autosomal dominant ichthyosis and X-linked ichthyosis. Comparison of their clinical and histological phenotypes. *Acta Derm Venereol*. 1991;71:431–434.

267. Hernández-Martín A, González-Sarmiento R, De Unamuno P. X-linked ichthyosis: an update. *Br J Dermatol*. 1999;141:617–627.

268. Zettersten E, Man MQ, Sato J, et al. Recessive x-linked ichthyosis: role of cholesterol-sulfate accumulation in the barrier abnormality. *J Invest Dermatol.* 1998;111:784–790.

269. Yang JM, Ahn KS, Cho MO, et al. Novel mutations of the transglutaminase 1 gene in lamellar ichthyosis. *J Invest Dermatol.* 2001;117:214–218.

270. Rothnagel JA, Dominey AM, Dempsey LD, et al. Mutations in the rod domains of keratins 1 and 10 in epidermolytic hyperkeratosis. *Science.* 1992;257:1128–1130.

271. el-Tonsy MH, el-Benhawi MO, Mehregan AH. Confluent and reticulated papillomatosis. *J Am Acad Dermatol.* 1987;16:893–894.

272. Lee SH, Choi EH, Lee WS, et al. Confluent and reticulated papillomatosis: a clinical, histopathological, and electron microscopic study. *J Dermatol.* 1991;18:725–730.

273. Panja RK. Acrokeratosis verruciformis: (Hopf)—a clinical entity? *Br J Dermatol.* 1977;96:643–652.

274. Dhitavat J, Macfarlane S, Dode L, et al. Acrokeratosis verruciformis of Hopf is caused by mutation in ATP2A2: evidence that it is allelic to Darier's disease. *J Invest Dermatol.* 2003;120:229–232.

275. Muller SA, Winkelmann RK. Alopecia areata. An evaluation of 736 patients. *Arch Dermatol.* 1963;88:290–297.

276. Elston DM, McCollough ML, Bergfeld WF, et al. Eosinophils in fibrous tracts and near hair bulbs: a helpful diagnostic feature of alopecia areata. *J Am Acad Dermatol.* 1997;37:101–106.

277. Sperling LC, Lupton GP. Histopathology of non-scarring alopecia. *J Cutan Pathol.* 1995;22:97–114.

278. Whiting DA. Possible mechanisms of miniaturization during androgenetic alopecia or pattern hair loss. *J Am Acad Dermatol.* 2001;45:S81–S86.

279. Muller SA. Trichotillomania: a histopathologic study in sixty-six patients. *J Am Acad Dermatol.* 1990;23:56–62.

280. Amato L, Mei S, Massi D, et al. Cicatricial alopecia; a dermatopathologic and immunopathologic study of 33 patients (pseudopelade of Brocq is not a specific clinico-pathologic entity). *Int J Dermatol.* 2002;41:8–15.

281. Dinehart SM, Herzberg AJ, Kerns BJ, et al. Acne keloidalis: a review. *J Dermatol Surg Oncol.* 1989;15:642–647.

282. Sperling LC, Homoky C, Pratt L, et al. Acne keloidalis is a form of primary scarring alopecia. *Arch Dermatol.* 2000;136:479–484.

283. Templeton SF, Solomon AR. Scarring alopecia: a classification based on microscopic criteria. *J Cutan Pathol.* 1994;21:97–109.

284. Gibson LE, Muller SA, Leiferman KM, et al. Follicular mucinosis: clinical and histopathologic study. *J Am Acad Dermatol.* 1989;20:441–446.

285. Gibson LE, Muller SA, Peters MS. Follicular mucinosis of childhood and adolescence. *Pediatr Dermatol.* 1988;5:231–235.

286. Barnett BO, Frieden IJ. Streptococcal skin diseases in children. *Semin Dermatol.* 1992;11:3–10.

287. Mancini AJ. Bacterial skin infections in children: the common and the not so common. *Pediatr Ann.* 2000;29:26–35.

288. Monday SR, Vath GM, Ferens WA, et al. Unique superantigen activity of staphylococcal exfoliative toxins. *J Immunol.* 1999;162:4550–4559.

289. Cribier B, Piemont Y, Grosshans E. Staphylococcal scalded skin syndrome in adults. A clinical review illustrated with a new case. *J Am Acad Dermatol.* 1994;30:319–324.

290. Frantzeskaki F, Betrosian AP. Ecthyma gangrenosum: a rare manifestation of Pseudomonas aeruginosa sepsis in a critically ill adult patient. *Eur J Dermatol.* 2008;18:345–346.

291. Kroshinsky D, Grossman ME, Fox LP. Approach to the patient with presumed cellulitis. *Semin Cutan Med Surg.* 2007;26:168–178.

292. Mohammed TT, Olumide YM. Chancroid and human immunodeficiency virus infection—a review. *Int J Dermatol.* 2008;47:1–8.

293. Hart G. Donovanosis. *Clin Infect Dis*. 1997;25:24–30; quiz 31–32.

294. Hart CA, Rao SK. Rhinoscleroma. *J Med Microbiol*. 2000;49:395–396.

295. Pardillo FE, Fajardo TT, Abalos RM, et al. Methods for the classification of leprosy for treatment purposes. *Clin Infect Dis*. 2007;44:1096–1099.

296. Cree IA, Coghill G, Subedi AM, et al. Effects of treatment on the histopathology of leprosy. *J Clin Pathol*. 1995;48:304–307.

297. Natrajan M, Katoch K, Katoch VM. Histology and immuno-histology of lesions clinically suspicious of leprosy. *Acta Leprol*. 1999;11:93–98.

298. Jeerapaet P, Ackerman AB. Histologic patterns of secondary syphilis. *Arch Dermatol*. 1973;107:373–377.

299. Abell E, Marks R, Jones EW. Secondary syphilis: a clinico-pathological review. *Br J Dermatol*. 1975;93:53–61.

300. Steere AC, Grodzicki RL, Kornblatt AN, et al. The spirochetal etiology of Lyme disease. *N Engl J Med*. 1983;308:733–740.

301. Berger BW. Erythema chronicum migrans of Lyme disease. *Arch Dermatol*. 1984;120:1017–1021.

302. Amsbaugh S, Huiras E, Wang NS, et al. Bacillary angiomatosis associated with pseudoepitheliomatous hyperplasia. *Am J Dermatopathol*. 2006;28:32–35.

303. Smith KJ, Skelton HG, Tuur S, et al. Bacillary angiomatosis in an immunocompetent child. *Am J Dermatopathol*. 1996;18:597–600.

304. Wong R, Tappero J, Cockerell CJ. Bacillary angiomatosis and other Bartonella species infections. *Semin Cutan Med Surg*. 1997;16:188–199.

305. Elewski BE, Hazen PG. The superficial mycoses and the dermatophytes. *J Am Acad Dermatol*. 1989;21:655–673.

306. Hebert AA. Tinea capitis: current concepts. *Arch Dermatol*. 1988;124:1554–1557.

307. Elewski BE. Tinea capitis: a current perspective. *J Am Acad Dermatol*. 2000;42:1–20; quiz 21–24.

308. Smith KJ, Neafie RC, Skelton HG III, et al. Majocchi's granuloma. *J Cutan Pathol*. 1991;18:28–35.

309. Macura AB. Dermatophyte infections. *Int J Dermatol*. 1993;32:313–323.

310. Silva-Lizama E. Tinea versicolor. *Int J Dermatol*. 1995;34:611–617.

311. Faergemann J, Fredriksson T. Tinea versicolor: some new aspects on etiology, pathogenesis, and treatment. *Int J Dermatol*. 1982;21:8–11.

312. Miles WJ, Branom WT Jr, Frank SB. Tinea nigra. Report of two cases and results of treatment with tolnaftate. *Arch Dermatol*. 1966;94:203–204.

313. Zaias N. Chromomycosis. *J Cutan Pathol*. 1978;5:155–164.

314. Minotto R, Bernardi CD, Mallmann LF, et al. Chromoblastomycosis: a review of 100 cases in the state of Rio Grande do Sul, Brazil. *J Am Acad Dermatol*. 2001;44:585–592.

315. McGinnis MR. Chromoblastomycosis and phaeohyphomycosis: new concepts, diagnosis, and mycology. *J Am Acad Dermatol*. 1983;8:1–16.

316. De Araujo T, Marques AC, Kerdel F. Sporotrichosis. *Int J Dermatol*. 2001;40:737–742.

317. Lurie HI. Histopathology of sporotrichosis. Notes on the nature of the asteroid body. *Arch Pathol*. 1963;75:421–437.

318. Fetter BF, Tindall JP. Cutaneous Sporotrichosis; Clinical study of nine cases utilizing an improved technique for demonstration of organisms. *Arch Pathol*. 1964;78:613–617.

319. Barfield L, Iacobelli D, Hashimoto K. Secondary cutaneous cryptococcosis: case report and review of 22 cases. *J Cutan Pathol*. 1988;15:385–392.

320. Dimino-Emme L, Gurevitch AW. Cutaneous manifestations of disseminated cryptococcosis. *J Am Acad Dermatol*. 1995;32:844–850.

321. Veglia KS, Marks VJ. Fusarium as a pathogen. A case report of Fusarium sepsis and review of the literature. *J Am Acad Dermatol*. 1987;16:260–263.

322. Bodey GP, Boktour M, Mays S, et al. Skin lesions associated with Fusarium infection. *J Am Acad Dermatol.* 2002;47:659–666.

323. Basler RS, Lagomarsino SL. Coccidioidomycosis: clinical review and treatment update. *Int J Dermatol.* 1979;18:104–110.

324. Stevens DA. Coccidioidomycosis. *N Engl J Med.* 1995;332:1077–1082.

325. DiCaudo DJ. Coccidioidomycosis: a review and update. *J Am Acad Dermatol.* 2006;55:929–942; quiz 943–945.

326. Hay RJ. Blastomycosis: what's new? *J Eur Acad Dermatol Venereol.* 2000;14:249–250.

327. Mason AR, Cortes GY, Cook J, et al. Cutaneous blastomycosis: a diagnostic challenge. *Int J Dermatol.* 2008;47:824–830.

328. Ramdial PK, Mosam A, Dlova NC, et al. Disseminated cutaneous histoplasmosis in patients infected with human immunodeficiency virus. *J Cutan Pathol.* 2002;29:215–225.

329. Eidbo J, Sanchez RL, Tschen JA, et al. Cutaneous manifestations of histoplasmosis in the acquired immune deficiency syndrome. *Am J Surg Pathol.* 1993;17:110–116.

330. Bonifaz A, Cansela R, Novales J, et al. Cutaneous histoplasmosis associated with acquired immunodeficiency syndrome (AIDS). *Int J Dermatol.* 2000;39:35–38.

331. Bakos L, Kronfeld M, Hampe S, et al. Disseminated paracoccidioidomycosis with skin lesions in a patient with acquired immunodeficiency syndrome. *J Am Acad Dermatol.* 1989;20:854–855.

332. Negroni R. Paracoccidioidomycosis (South American blastomycosis, Lutz's mycosis). *Int J Dermatol.* 1993;32:847–859.

333. Marchevsky AM, Bottone EJ, Geller SA, et al. The changing spectrum of disease, etiology, and diagnosis of mucormycosis. *Hum Pathol.* 1980;11:457–464.

334. Weinberg JM, Baxt RD, Egan CL, et al. Mucormycosis in a patient with acquired immunodeficiency syndrome. *Arch Dermatol.* 1997;133:249–251.

335. Cahill KM, Mofty AM, Kawaguchi TP. Primary cutaneous aspergillosis. *Arch Dermatol.* 1967;96:545–547.

336. Munn S, Keane F, Child F, et al. Primary cutaneous aspergillosis. *Br J Dermatol.* 1999;141:378–380.

337. Roilides E, Farmaki E. Human immunodeficiency virus infection and cutaneous aspergillosis. *Arch Dermatol.* 2000;136:412–414.

338. Date A, Ramakrishna B, Lee VN, et al. Tumoral rhinosporidiosis. *Histopathology.* 1995;27:288–290.

339. Ghorpade A. Giant cutaneous rhinosporidiosis. *J Eur Acad Dermatol Venereol.* 2006;20:88–89.

340. Rodríguez-Toro G. Lobomycosis. *Int J Dermatol.* 1993;32:324–332.

341. Tapia A, Torres-Calcindo A, Arosemena R. Keloidal blastomycosis (Lobo's disease) in Panama. *Int J Dermatol.* 1978;17:572–574.

342. Jaramillo D, Cortes A, Restrepo A, et al. Lobomycosis. Report of the eighth Colombian case and review of the literature. *J Cutan Pathol.* 1976;3:180–189.

343. Nebesio CL, Mirowski GW, Chuang TY. Human papillomavirus: clinical significance and malignant potential. *Int J Dermatol.* 2001;40:373–379.

344. Young R, Jolley D, Marks R. Comparison of the use of standardized diagnostic criteria and intuitive clinical diagnosis in the diagnosis of common viral warts (verrucae vulgaris). *Arch Dermatol.* 1998;134:1586–1589.

345. Steigleder GK. Histology of benign virus induced tumors of the skin. *J Cutan Pathol.* 1978;5:45–52.

346. Berger TG, Sawchuk WS, Leonardi C, et al. Epidermodysplasia verruciformis-associated papillomavirus infection complicating human immunodeficiency virus disease. *Br J Dermatol.* 1991;124:79–83.

347. Rock B, Shah KV, Farmer ER. A morphologic, pathologic, and virologic study of anogenital warts in men. *Arch Dermatol.* 1992;128:495–500.

348. Sykes NL Jr. Condyloma acuminatum. *Int J Dermatol*. 1995;34:297–302.
349. Fatahzadeh M, Schwartz RA. Human herpes simplex virus infections: epidemiology, pathogenesis, symptomatology, diagnosis, and management. *J Am Acad Dermatol*. 2007;57:737–763; quiz 764–766.
350. Fatahzadeh M, Schwartz RA. Human herpes simplex labialis. *Clin Exp Dermatol*. 2007;32:625–630.
351. McSorley J, Shapiro L, Brownstein MH, et al. Herpes simplex and varicella-zoster: comparative histopathology of 77 cases. *Int J Dermatol*. 1974;13:69–75.
352. Martin JR, Holt RK, Langston C, et al. Type-specific identification of herpes simplex and varicella-zoster virus antigen in autopsy tissues. *Hum Pathol*. 1991;22:75–80.
353. Cribier B, Scrivener Y, Grosshans E. Molluscum contagiosum: histologic patterns and associated lesions. A study of 578 cases. *Am J Dermatopathol*. 2001;23:99–103.
354. Gottlieb SL, Myskowski PL. Molluscum contagiosum. *Int J Dermatol*. 1994;33:453–461.
355. Johannessen JV, Krogh HK, Solberg I, et al. Human orf. *J Cutan Pathol*. 1975;2:265–283.
356. Gill MJ, Arlette J, Buchan KA, et al. Human orf. A diagnostic consideration? *Arch Dermatol*. 1990;126:356–358.
357. Sanchez RL, Hebert A, Lucia H, et al. Orf. A case report with histologic, electron microscopic, and immunoperoxidase studies. *Arch Pathol Lab Med*. 1985;109:166–170.
358. Leavell UW Jr, Phillips IA. Milker's nodules. Pathogenesis, tissue culture, electron microscopy, and calf inoculation. *Arch Dermatol*. 1975;111:1307–1311.
359. Groves RW, Wilson-Jones E, MacDonald DM. Human orf and milkers' nodule: a clinicopathologic study. *J Am Acad Dermatol*. 1991;25:706–711.
360. Lee S, Kim KY, Hahn CS, et al. Gianotti-Crosti syndrome associated with hepatitis B surface antigen (subtype adr). *J Am Acad Dermatol*. 1985;12:629–633.
361. Taieb A, Plantin P, Du Pasquier P, et al. Gianotti-Crosti syndrome: a study of 26 cases. *Br J Dermatol*. 1986;115:49–59.
362. Caputo R, Gelmetti C, Ermacora E, et al. Gianotti-Crosti syndrome: a retrospective analysis of 308 cases. *J Am Acad Dermatol*. 1992;26:207–210.
363. Alacoque B, Cloppet H, Dumontel C, et al. Histological, immunofluorescent, and ultrastructural features of lymphogranuloma venereum: a case report. *Br J Vener Dis*. 1984;60:390–395.
364. Kapoor S. Re-emergence of lymphogranuloma venereum. *J Eur Acad Dermatol Venereol*. 2008;22:409–416.
365. Akilov OE, Khachemoune A, Hasan T. Clinical manifestations and classification of Old World cutaneous leishmaniasis. *Int J Dermatol*. 2007;46:132–142.
366. Samady JA, Schwartz RA. Old World cutaneous leishmaniasis. *Int J Dermatol*. 1997;36:161–166.
367. Azulay RD, Azulay DR Jr. Immune-clinical-pathologic spectrum of leishmaniasis. *Int J Dermatol*. 1995;34:303–307.
368. Sangueza OP, Sangueza JM, Stiller MJ, et al. Mucocutaneous leishmaniasis: a clinicopathologic classification. *J Am Acad Dermatol*. 1993;28:927–932.
369. High WA, Bravo FG. Emerging diseases in tropical dermatology. *Adv Dermatol*. 2007;23:335–350.
370. Cho BK, Ham SH, Lee JY, et al. Cutaneous protothecosis. *Int J Dermatol*. 2002;41:304–306.
371. Sudman MS. Protothecosis. A critical review. *Am J Clin Pathol*. 1974;61:10–19.
372. Mendez CM, Silva-Lizama E, Logemann H. Human cutaneous protothecosis. *Int J Dermatol*. 1995;34:554–555.
373. Amatya BM, Kimula Y. Cysticercosis in Nepal: a histopathologic study of sixty-two cases. *Am J Surg Pathol*. 1999;23:1276–1279.
374. Uthida-Tanaka AM, Sampaio MC, Velho PE, et al. Subcutaneous and cerebral cysticercosis. *J Am Acad Dermatol*. 2004;50:S14–S17.

375. Gutierrez Y. Diagnostic features of zoonotic filariae in tissue sections. *Hum Pathol.* 1984;15:514–525.

376. Payan HM. Human infection with Dirofilaria. *Arch Dermatol.* 1978;114:593–594.

377. Pampiglione S, Rivasi F, Angeli G, et al. Dirofilariasis due to Dirofilaria repens in Italy, an emergent zoonosis: report of 60 new cases. *Histopathology.* 2001;38:344–354.

378. Angeli L, Tiberio R, Zuccoli R, et al. Human dirofilariasis: 10 new cases in Piedmont, Italy. *Int J Dermatol.* 2007;46:844–847.

379. Connor DH, Williams PH, Helwig EB, et al. Dermal changes in onchocerciasis. *Arch Pathol.* 1969;87:193–200.

380. Connor DH, George GH, Gibson DW. Pathologic changes of human onchocerciasis: implications for future research. *Rev Infect Dis.* 1985;7:809–819.

381. Okulicz JF, Stibich AS, Elston DM, et al. Cutaneous onchocercoma. *Int J Dermatol.* 2004;43:170–172.

382. Caumes E, Ly F, Bricaire F. Cutaneous larva migrans with folliculitis: report of seven cases and review of the literature. *Br J Dermatol.* 2002;146:314–316.

383. Blackwell V, Vega-Lopez F. Cutaneous larva migrans: clinical features and management of 44 cases presenting in the returning traveller. *Br J Dermatol.* 2001;145:434–437.

384. Jucowics P, Ramon ME, Don PC, et al. Norwegian scabies in an infant with acquired immunodeficiency syndrome. *Arch Dermatol.* 1989;125:1670–1671.

385. Falk ES, Eide TJ. Histologic and clinical findings in human scabies. *Int J Dermatol.* 1981;20:600–605.

386. Fernandez N, Torres A, Ackerman AB. Pathologic findings in human scabies. *Arch Dermatol.* 1977;113:320–324.

387. Sanusi ID, Brown EB, Shepard TG, et al. Tungiasis: report of one case and review of the 14 reported cases in the United States. *J Am Acad Dermatol.* 1989;20:941–944.

388. Wentzell JM, Schwartz BK, Pesce JR. Tungiasis. *J Am Acad Dermatol.* 1986;15:117–119.

Index

NOTE: *Page numbers followed by 'f' indicate figures.*